LEAD POISONING IN MAN AND THE ENVIRONMENT

Papers by

Eva L. Jernigan, John L. Bové, J.C. Langford, Robert S. Morse, P.J. Magno, R.L. Blanchard, L.U. Joshi, Clair C. Patterson, Robert G. Oliver, Vilma R. Hunt, R.E. Stanley, G.D. Potter, L. Kostial, K.M. Scott, Thomas Murphy, S. Hernberg, Brana Jovičić, W.A.M. den Tonkelaar, Sverre H. Omang, D.M. Groffman, Harry Levine, N.J. Prakash, James W. Sayre, et al.

MSS Information Corporation
655 Madison Avenue, New York, N.Y. 10021

Library of Congress Cataloging in Publication Data
Main entry under title:

Lead poisoning in man and the environment.

    1. Lead-poisoning--Addresses, essays, lectures.
2. Environmental health--Addresses, essays, lectures.
I. Jernigan, Eva L. [DNLM: 1. Environmental health
--Collected works. 2. Lead poisoning--Collected works.
QV 292 L434 1973]
RA1231.L4L4 1973   615.9'25'68808   72-13817
ISBN 0-8422-7105-8

TABLE OF CONTENTS

CREDITS AND ACKNOWLEDGEMENTS

Blanchard, R.L.; and J.B. Moore, " ^{210}Pb and ^{210}Po in Tissues of Some Alaskan Residents as Related to Consumption of Caribou or Reindeer Meat," *Health Physics*, 1970, 18:127-134.

Blanchard, R.L.; and J.B. Moore, "Body Burden, Distribution and Internal Dose of ^{210}Pb and ^{210}Po in a Uranium Miner Population," *Health Physics*, 1971, 21:499-518.

Bové, John L.; and Stanley Siebenberg, "Airborne Lead and Carbon Monoxide at 45th Street, New York City," *Science*, 1970, 167:986-987.

Groffman, D.M.; and R. Wood, "Revision of a Field Method for the Determination of Total Airborne Lead," *Analyst*, 1971, 96:140-145.

Hernberg, S.; and J. Nikkanen, "Enzyme Inhibition by Lead Under Normal Urban Conditions," *Lancet*, 1970, 1:63-64.

Hunt, V.R., "Concentrations of ^{210}Po, ^{226}Ra and ^{228}Th in the Choroid of the Eye, Particularly in Cattle," *Radioecological Concentration Processes*, 1966, 303-311.

Hunt, Vilma R.; Edward P. Radford, Jr.; and Ascher Segall, "Naturally Occurring Concentrations of Alpha-Emitting Isotopes in a New England Population," *Health Physics*, 1970, 19:235-243.

Jernigan, Eva L.; Barbara J. Ray; and Robert A. Duce, "Lead and Bromine in Atmospheric Particulate Matter on Oahu, Hawaii," *Atmospheric Environment*, 1971, 5:881-886.

Joshi, L.U.; and T.N. Mahadevan, "Seasonal Variations of Radium-D (Lead-210) in Ground Level Air in India," *Health Physics*, 1968, 15:67-71.

Joshi, L.U.; C. Rangarajan; and Sarada Gopalakrishnan, "Measurements of Lead-210 in Surface Air and Precipitation," *Health Physics*, 1969, 21:107-112.

Joshi, L.U.; C. Rangarajan; and Sarada Gopalakrishnan, "Investigations on ^{210}Pb Concentrations in Various Regions of India," *Health Physics*, 1971, 20:665-668.

Jovičić, Brana, "Ulcer and Gastritis in the Professions Exposed to Lead," *Archives of Environmental Health*, 1970, 21:526-528.

Kostial, L.; I. Šimonović; and M. Pišonić, "Reduction of Lead Absorption from the Intestine in Newborn Rats," *Environmental Research*, 1971, 4:360-363.

Langford, J.C., "Particulate Pb, ^{210}Pb and ^{210}Po in the Environment," *Health Physics*, 1971, 20:331-336.

Levine, Harry; and Paul S. Ruggera, "A Field Method for the Determination of Lead in Glass Used for Shielding Television Receiver

Components," *American Industrial Hygiene Association Journal*, 1970, 31:633-636.

Magno, P.J.; P.R. Groulx; and J.C. Apidianakis, "Lead-210 in Air and Total Diets in the United States During 1966," *Health Physics*, 1970, 18:383-388.

Morse, Robert S.; and George A. Welford, "Dietary Intake of ^{210}Pb," *Health Physics*, 1971, 21:53-55.

Murphy, Thomas; and Martha L. Lepow, "Comparison of Delta-Aminolevulinic Acid Levels in Urine and Blood Lead Levels for Screening Children for Lead Poisoning," *Connecticut Medicine*, 1971, 35: 488-492.

Oliver, Robert G., "Lead and the Legislature — 1971," *Connecticut Medicine*, 1971, 35:498-500.

Omang, Sverre H., "The Determination of Lead in Air by Flameless Atomic Absorption Spectrophotometry," *Analytica Chimica Acta*, 1971, 55:439-441.

Patterson, Clair C., "Lead in the Environment," *Connecticut Medicine*, 1971, 35:347-352.

Potter, G.D.; D.R. McIntyre; and G.M. Vattuone, "The Fate and Implications of [203]Pb Ingestion in a Dairy Cow and a Calf," *Health Physics*, 1971, 20:650-653.

Prakash, N.J.; and W.W. Harrison, "A Simple Demountable Hollow-Cathode Tube for the Analysis of Solutions: Application to Lead in Biological Materials," *Analytica Chimica Acta*, 1971, 53:421-427.

Sayre, James W.; and David J. Wilson, "A Spot Test for Detection of Lead in Paint," *Pediatrics*, 1970, 46:783-785.

Scott, K.M.; K.M. Hwang; M. Jurkowitz; and G.P. Brierley, "Ion Transport by Heart Mitochondria: XXIII. The Effects of Lead on Mitochondrial Reactions," *Archives of Biochemistry and Biophysics*, 1971, 147:557-567.

Stanley, R.E.; A.A. Mullen; and E.W. Bretthauer, "Transfer to Milk of Ingested Radiolead," *Health Physics*, 1971, 21:211-215.

Tonkelaar, W.A.M. Den; and Martha A. Bikker, "Microdetermination of Lead on Tapes of an A.I.S.I. Automatic Air Sampler by Atomic Absorption Spectroscopy," *Atmospheric Environment*, 1971, 5:353-356.

PREFACE

This is the first of two volumes of collected papers dealing with lead poisoning in man. This volume which contains reports published from 1970-1972, focusses on the presence of lead in the atmosphere, the soil, water, plants, and hence in the food eaten by humans. Papers concerning the effects of lead metabolites on cellular systems and on occupational exposure to toxic levels of lead are included. A major portion of this volume is devoted to new methods for the analytical detection of lead in biological samples as well as other materials involved in the epidemiology of lead poisoning, such as paint.

This two-volume series on *Lead* represents another addition to the MSS library of readings in ecology.

Lead In The Environment: Atmosphere

LEAD AND BROMINE IN ATMOSPHERIC PARTICULATE MATTER ON OAHU, HAWAII

EVA L. JERNIGAN
BARBARA J. RAY
and
ROBERT A. DUCE

INTRODUCTION

THERE has been very little work published on the relationship between atmospheric particulate lead and bromine originating from the burning of leaded gasoline. LININGER et al. (1966) point out that the ethyl fluid mixture of tetraethyllead, ethylene dibromide, and ethylene dichloride has the weight ratios Pb:Br:Cl of 1.00:0.39:0.34 with about 2–3 g of lead present in each gallon of gasoline. HIRSCHLER et al. (1957, 1964) studied the chemical composition of automobile exhaust, using an electrostatic precipitator and X-ray diffraction analysis and found the following compounds: $PbCl \cdot Br$, $\alpha NH_4Cl \cdot 2PbCl \cdot Br$, $\beta NH_4Cl \cdot 2PbCl \cdot Br$, $2NH_4Cl \cdot PbCl \cdot Br$, $PbO \cdot PSO_4$, and $PbO \cdot PbCl \cdot Br \cdot H_2O$. The predominant species was found to be the double salt $PbCl \cdot Br$ which also has a weight ratio Pb:Cl:Br of 1.00:0.39:0.34.

LININGER et al. (1966) corrected the particulate bromine concentration observed in the atmosphere in the Boston area for a natural component due to sea salt and called the resulting Br concentration "excess Br". They then calculated "excess Br"/Pb ratios which varied from 0.006 to 0.54, averaging 0.21 ± 0.16, with only one of the ten samples having an excess Br/Pb ratio greater than the ethyl fluid ratio of 0.39. There appeared to be a correlation between the excess Br/Pb ratio and visibility, higher visibility being associated with lower ratios. LININGER et al. (1966) suggested these results indicated that after the lead halide particles are exhausted into the atmosphere, some of the Br is released from the particles by chemical reactions. They further suggested that on hazy days these reactions might be inhibited, perhaps due to the condensation of water vapor on the particles and the consequent reduction of the intensity of solar radiation.

WINCHESTER et al. (1967) studied this problem further in Fairbanks, Alaska in the winter. This site was far from the complicating influence of the sea, and it was expected that the low temperatures and low intensity of ultraviolet light might inhibit the release of Br from the particles. The excess Br/Pb ratios averaged 0.15 ± 0.08 for sixteen curbside samples in Fairbanks. The excess Cl/Pb ratio was 0.36 ± 0.10, very close to the ethyl fluid ratio of 0.34, consistent with the view that the initially formed lead halide aerosol has the same relative composition as the ethyl fluid itself. WINCHESTER et al. (1967) concluded that since a pronounced Br deficiency is observed both in Massachusetts and in Alaska in the winter, neither temperature nor light intensity may be important variables in determining the loss of Br from the particles. They further suggested that oxidation of Br^- to Br_2 by ozone might cause the release. PIERRARD (1969), however, has studied the photochemical dissociation of PbBrCl in carbon tetrachloride in the laboratory. His results indicate that both Br_2 and Cl_2 are released by photolysis of PbBrCl and he expects the same type of reaction will occur in the ambient polluted atmosphere. He further states that the dependence of the excess Br/Pb ratio on visibility in the work of LININGER et al. (1966) can be explained by the reduction of shorter wavelength solar radiation by the haze particles.

The present investigation was undertaken for two reasons. The first was to determine the excess Br/Pb ratio in particulate matter in the atmosphere over Honolulu. When compared to the studies made in Massachusetts and Alaska, this information might show the effect of higher environmental temperatures and the intensity of solar radiation on the possible chemical reactions responsible for the loss of bromine from the particles.

Second, the amount of lead and bromine in the atmosphere in Hawaii can be used as an index to estimate the relative amount of automotive pollution experienced in Honolulu through comparison with levels found in other cities in the United States. Meteorologically, Hawaii is under the influence of the northeast tradewinds, especially during the summer when they are particularly well-developed. During normal tradewind conditions, the base of the tradewind inversion is approximately 2000 m above sea level and winds from the east northeast predominate, with speed generally 2–10 m s^{-1} (LEOPOLD, 1951). The citizens of Hawaii have assumed, until recently, that the tradewinds carry Honolulu's air pollution rapidly out to sea before it has time to build up to significant levels. In this work, samples were taken along the sidewalks of urban Honolulu, in the summer of 1968 during normal tradewind conditions, to determine the levels of pollution at ground level.

Honolulu is particularly well-suited for a study of this type since it is isolated from the mainland and is thus far from pollution sources which could contribute pollutants not originating in the area under consideration. CHOW et al. (1969) have shown that lead concentrations over the Pacific Ocean far from the North American continent are negligible in comparison with the values found in this study, even in relatively unpolluted locations in Hawaii. This has been corroborated by HOFFMAN (1971). It can be safely assumed, therefore, that essentially all the pollution aerosols found in Hawaii originate in Hawaii. Approximately 41×10^6 gal of gasoline were sold on Oahu during June, July, and August of 1968 when the samples in this study were collected (STATE OF HAWAII, 1969) and virtually all gasoline sold in Hawaii contains tetraethyl-lead in concentrations up to 3.1 g gal $^{-1}$ (HEU, 1969). Ethyl fluid is probably also the primary source of bromine in urban Hawaii. DUCE et al. (1965) report that the maximum concentration of bromine in unpolluted marine air over the island of Hawaii is approximately $0.02 \ \mu g \ m^{-3}$. In comparison with the values of bromine found in urban areas in this study, this contribution is very small indeed.

EXPERIMENTAL

Sampling procedures

(i) *Apparatus.* Samples were collected on 8 in. × 10 in. glass fiber filters (Gelman Type A, without organic binder). The filters were mounted on Gelman Hurricane high volume pumps (Model 16003) at high speed with no orifice, giving a flow rate of $200 \pm 20 \ m^3 \ h^{-1}$. The pump was powered in the field by a gasoline driven generator. Care was always taken to locate the generator downwind from the pump and filter. Two simultaneous samples were taken at each location with both pumps one meter above the ground and the filter oriented into the wind. Samples were taken over a 4-h period (800 m^3) in heavily polluted areas and over an 8-h period (1600 m^3) in relatively unpolluted areas. All samples were taken during daylight hours. Filters were dismounted in the field and placed in polyethylene bags which were sealed and placed in a freezer to prevent loss of more volatile components. Samples were analyzed within a year after collection. According to the manufacturer, these filters have collection efficiencies of $\geq$ 99.7 per cent for particles with diameters $>$ 0.3 μm and $>$ 98 per cent for particles with a diameter of 0.05 μm. Robinson and Ludwig (1968) report that the mean mass equivalent diameter (MMED) of lead particles in urban air is approximately 0.25 μm, while LEE et al. (1969) find that the MMED is approximately 0.2 μm. In the present study, a test was made to determine what mass fraction of the lead passed through the glass fiber filter. A 47 mm dia. 0.1 μm pore diameter Millipore filter was mounted in a filter holder behind a Type A glass fiber filter of the same size, and a sample was collected at the parking garage location (see below). Seven per cent of the mass of particulate lead penetrated the glass fiber filter and was collected on the Millipore filter. From the results of this test and the information supplied by the manufacturer, it is believed that at least 90–95 per cent of the mass of particulate lead was collected on the glass fiber filters used in this study.

(ii) *Collection sites.* Sampling sites in the Honolulu area were divided into several classes: a parking garage—urban curbsides—urban roofs, parks and open parking lots—rural interior and leeward sites—and rural windward coastal sites. The parking garage was at the Ala Moana Shopping Center, which has parking on 3 levels. Samples were taken on all three levels. The curbside locations were primarily in commercial areas. The filter and pump were generally placed downwind of the street or intersection, 2–4 m from the curb. Other urban locations included parking lots, parks, and roofs. The roof locations were at the University of Hawaii (4 story building) in a residential area, and at the Pearl Harbor Weather Station (3 story building) adjacent to a major highway. The rural sites were located far from major highways—in pineapple fields, on mountain slopes, and on beaches.

At all collection sites, the wind speed and direction humidity, temperature, and traffic count were recorded at least once every hour. Generally, meteorological conditions were quite constant, typical of the well-developed northeast tradewind system during the summer months.

Analytical procedures

(i) *Elution procedure.* Each filter sample was cut into four equal parts. Each part was eluted with 25.0 ml of 0.1 N HNO_3. Blanks, run on clean filters eluted with this same acid, yielded values less than

11

0.2 ppm Pb and 0.04 ppm Br in the extracting solution and constituted less than 10 per cent of the sample, even for relatively unpolluted samples. Six-normal HNO_3 yielded higher blank values for Pb and was no more effective in removing the particles from the filters than the 0.1 N HNO_3. The filter and eluting acid were placed in a Branson ultrasonic cleaner for 10 min to remove the particulate matter from the filter. Studies showed that ultrasonic cleaning reached a maximum efficiency after 5 min. Cleaning times greater than 5 min produced no variation in the amount of lead or bromine eluted from the filters. Subsequent washings with fresh acid and further ultrasonic cleaning showed that 98 per cent of the particulate lead was removed from the filter in the first extraction. The solutions were then decanted from the filter and placed in acid washed polyethylene containers for analysis. The solutions were analyzed for Pb within 4 h of elution to prevent loss of Pb due to adsorption on the polyethylene containers.

(ii) *Lead analysis*. The solutions were analyzed for Pb by atomic absorption spectroscopy, using a Perkin–Elmer Model 303 double beam atomic absorption spectrophotometer equipped with a 3 slot Boling burning using an acetylene-air flame and an Intensitron hollow cathode lead lamp. The 2170 Å line, being more sensitive in aqueous solutions than the 2883 Å line, was used in this study. The precision of the analyses was 0.2 ppm, the sensitivity was 0.3 ppm, and the detection limit in aqueous solution was 0.2 ppm, in accordance with definitions by KAHN (1968). For further details on the lead analyses, see JERNIGAN (1969).

(iii) *Bromide analysis*. Bromide was determined using a specific ion electrode of the solid silver halide type, Orion Ionalyzer Bromide Ion Activity Electrode, Model 94–53. The bromide electrode was operated using a Beckman Expandomatic pH meter in the expanded scale mode. The instrument is reproducible to $\pm$ 0.3 mV in this mode, and with frequent calibration, the electrode gives readings which are reproducible to $\pm$ 1 per cent of the bromide activity in the sample. The reference electrode used was the Orion Model 90–02 Double Junction Reference Electrode. It is estimated that the overall precision of the Br analyses is $\pm$ 0.05 ppm Br. For further details concerning the bromide analysis see RAY (1969).

RESULTS AND DISCUSSION

A summary of the Pb and Br concentrations found in Honolulu as a function of sampling location is presented in TABLE 1. Concentrations determined for individual samples are not reported to conserve space. These data, as well as meteorological information for these samples, will be furnished to the interested reader on request.

The only other atmospheric lead values available for Honolulu were collected as part of the National Air Sampling Network (NASN) from the roof of the Board of Health building in downtown Honolulu. The NASN samples show lead concentrations ranging between 0.16 and 0.8 μg m^{-3} during June and July, 1968 (ENRIONE, 1971). These values compare well with values of lead found during the same period at urban roofs and parking lots in the present study. Curbside concentrations of Pb found in Honolulu approximate levels found in other U.S. cities. The average curbside value for lead found in this study was 7.7 μg m^{-3}, which approaches the average Pb concentration found along the streets of downtown Los Angeles at similar periods of the day, 10.5 μg m^{-3} (KONOPINSKI et al., 1967). The

TABLE 1. SUMMARY OF Pb AND Br CONCENTRATIONS OBTAINED IN HONOLULU, HAWAII

Type of location	No. of sites	No. of samples	Pb concentration* (μg m^{-3})			Br concentration* (μg m^{-3})		
			Min.	Max.	Mean	Min.	Max.	Mean
Parking garage	3	12	2.10	29.0	12.45	0.49	10.50	3.83
Urban curbsides	9	31	2.00	13.8	7.73	0.36	3.50	1.60
Other urban (parks, roofs, and parking lots)	10	30	0.08	6.10	1.64	0.026	1.31	0.35
Rural—interior and leeward	3	5	0.08	0.29	0.23	0.12	0.17	0.15
Rural—windward	1	2	0.0017	0.0017	0.0017	0.81	0.81	0.81

* Overall uncertainty in Pb and Br concentrations $\pm$ 12 per cent.

mean Pb content for cities in Honolulu's population class is 1.2 μg m^{-3} (Ludwig *et al.*, 1970). This data, taken from the NASN, was derived generally from roofs of buildings in downtown areas. The present study showed roof values of Pb near an intersection averaging 1.5 μg m^{-3}, approximating the national average.

The highest concentration of atmospheric Pb observed in this study, 29 μg m^{-3}, was found at the Ala Moana Shopping Center underground parking garage, characterized by very poor circulation. The highest curbside concentration of lead, 23.5 μg m^{-3}, was found at the Wilson Tunnel through the Koolau Mountains, also characterized by poor circulation. This concentration is considerably higher than the maximum concentration of Pb found in outlet air from Sumner Tunnel, Boston, where a value of 9 μg m^{-3} was obtained (Conlee *et al.*, 1967). No values as high as the 40 μg m^{-3} reported on Los Angeles freeways (Konopinski *et al.*, 1967) were found in Honolulu.

All the bromide values obtained in this study exceeded the values found by Duce *et al.* (1965) in the unpolluted marine atmosphere around the island of Hawaii (0.01–0.02 μg m^{-3} for windward land stations, 0.001–0.01 μg m^{-3} for aircraft samples over the sea). However, several values at roof and park locations were found to be in the range reported in Fairbanks, Alaska (0.021–0.065 μg m^{-3}). Previous to this study, the highest value observed for atmospheric particulate bromine was 1.38 μg m^{-3} found in pollution aerosols of Calumet Harbour, Michigan (Loucks *et al.*, 1969). The mean curbside value found in this study was 1.60 μg m^{-3} with a maximum curbside value of 3.5 μg m^{-3}, somewhat higher than previous measurements of atmospheric bromine in cities.

The maximum bromide concentration of 10.50 μg m^{-3} was found at the Ala Moana Shopping Center's basement garage. The Wilson Tunnel location yielded a high value of 6.00 μg m^{-3}.

Excess bromine values, after Lininger *et al.* (1966), can be calculated according to equation (1):

$$\text{Excess Br} = \text{Total Br} - \text{Sea salt Br} \tag{1}$$

A maximum value for particulate sea salt Br over land in Hawaii was found to be 0.02 μg m^{-3} (Duce *et al.*, 1965). This value for the sea salt bromine contribution represents only a small fraction of the total bromine observed for over 95 per cent of the samples in this study, even in relatively unpolluted locations. Thus, the excess bromine is essentially the same as the total particulate bromide concentration in this work.

Perhaps the most striking result is the relationship found between the lead and bromide values in pollution aerosols in Honolulu. Figure 1 presents a plot of total particulate bromide vs. particulate lead concentrations for all samples collected at outdoor curbside and parking lot locations in Honolulu. A least squares regression line through these points is also presented in Fig. 1. The slope of this line (Br/Pb) is 0.22 and the coefficient of correlation between bromide and lead is 0.97. Also illustrated

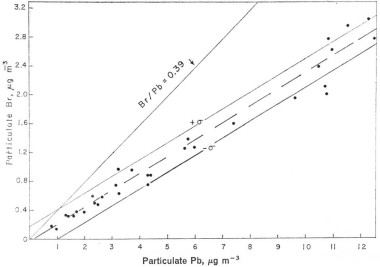

Fig. 1. Particulate lead vs. particulate bromide concentrations for urban curbside and parking lot samples in Honolulu, Hawaii.

13

on FIG. 1 is a line with slope Br/Pb = 0.39, which represents the ratio of Br/Pb in ethyl fluid. This line also represents the Br/Pb ratio found in the predominant exhaust species containing lead, $PbCl.Br$. If there were no reactions involving loss of bromine from these particles, the Br/Pb ratio found in pollution aerosols should be 0.39. In this study, similar to the work in Alaska and Massachusetts, the observed Br/Pb ratio is considerably less than 0.39.

The average Br/Pb ratio for outdoor curbside and parking lot samples in this study, 0.22 ± 0.04, agrees with the average ratio found by LININGER *et al.* (1966) in Massachusetts, 0.21 ± 0.16, but is somewhat higher than the average ratio found by WINCHESTER *et al.* (1967) in Alaska, 0.15 ± 0.08. Clearly, the previous investigations show considerable scatter in the Br/Pb ratios; whereas, the ratios are remarkably consistent in the present study. This constancy in the Br/Pb ratio is probably due to the persistent meteorological conditions found in Hawaii during the summer months. The temperature during curbside sampling in the summer of 1968 ranged between 26 and 33°C, the relative humidity between 53 and 75 per cent, and the winds were primarily from the east northeast at velocities between 1–6 m s^{-1}. There were no periods of haze or fog, as were observed in the Massachusetts and Alaskan studies, and all samples were collected during the daytime.

The regression line in FIG. 1 passes through the origin, strongly supporting the belief that in polluted air, lead and bromide originate from the same source—automobiles. This also indicates that the sea salt contribution to the bromide concentration is not significant in Honolulu, even though the city is surrounded by this potential source.

CONCLUSIONS

(1) The atmospheric particulate Br/Pb ratios found in this study are lower than the ethyl fluid ratio 0.39, and are quite constant, averaging 0.22 ± 0.04. The constancy is probably due to the persistent meteorological conditions characteristics of the tradewind regime. For example, marked variations in solar radiation intensity due to variations in cloud cover, haze, and nocturnal and diurnal sampling were minimal in this study, in contrast to previous studies in Massachusetts and Alaska. The effect of the higher ambient temperature in Hawaii compared to winter Alaska appears to be a relatively unimportant factor in the loss of Br from the particles. A detailed study of the variation of the Br/Pb ratio with particle size would be a significant aid in understanding the possible release of gaseous Br from these particles, especially if the various lead containing compounds are found in different size fractions.

(2) Honolulu has a very significant problem with automotive air pollution. All of the samples represented on FIG. 1 were obtained under normal tradewind conditions and, therefore, represent atmospheric lead and bromine concentrations during periods when there should be maximum dispersion of pollutants. Even under these conditions, ground level pollution lead and bromide concentrations are similar or higher than those found in other cities in the United States.

Acknowledgements—We would like to thank GERALD L. HOFFMAN, University of Hawaii, for aid in the atomic absorption analyses. This work was supported in part by the Environmental Protection Agency, Air Pollution Control Office, under grant R01 AP 00617-2.

REFERENCES

CHOW T. J., EARL J. L. and BENNENT C. F. (1969) Lead aerosols in marine atmosphere. *Environ. Sci. Technol.* **3**, 737–740.

CONLEE C. J., KENLINE P. A., CUMMINS R. L. and KONOPINSKI V. J. (1967) Motor vehicle exhaust at three selected sites. *Archs environ. Hlth* **14**, 429–446.

DUCE R. A., WINCHESTER J. W. and VAN NAHL T. (1965) Iodine, bromine, and chlorine in the Hawaiian marine atmosphere. *J. geophys. Res.* **70**, 1775–1779.

ENRIONE R. E. (1971) Metals and Advanced Analysis Lab, National Air Surveillance Network, Environmental Protection Agency, Cincinnati, Ohio. Personal communication.

HEU K. (1969) Standard Oil of California, Hawaiian Refinery. Personal communication.

HIRSCHLER D. A., GILBERT L. F., LAMB F. W. and NIEBYLSKI L. M. (1957) Particulate lead compounds in automobile exhaust gas. *Ind. engng Chem.* **49**, 1131–1142.

HIRSCHLER D. A. and GILBERT L. F. (1964) Nature of lead in automobile exhaust gas. *Archs environ. Hlth* **8**, 109–125.

HOFFMAN G. L. (1971) Ph.D. dissertation, Department of Chemistry, University of Hawaii.

JERNIGAN E. L. (1969) M. S. thesis, Department of Chemistry, University of Hawaii.

KAHN H. L. (1968) *Atomic Absorption Spectroscopy, Trace Inorganics in Water*, Advances in Chemistry Series, edited by R. F. GOULD, No. 73, pp. 183–229. American Chemical Society.

KONOPINSKI V. J. and UPHAM J. B. (1967) Commuter exposure to atmospheric lead. *Archs environ. Hlth.* **14**, 589–593.

LEE R. E., JR., PATTERSON R. K. and WAGMAN J. (1968) Particle size distribution of metal components in urban air. *Environ. Sci. Technol.* **2**, 288–290.

LEOPOLD L. B. (1951) Hawaiian climate: its relation to human and plant geography. *Meteorol. Monogr.* **1**, (3), 1–6.

LININGER R. L., DUCE R. A., WINCHESTER J. W. and MATSON W. R. (1966) Chlorine, bromine, iodine and lead in aerosols from Cambridge, Massachusetts. *J. geophys. Res.* **71**, 2457–2463.

LOUCKS R. H., WINCHESTER J. W., MATSON W. R. and TIFFANY M. A. (1969) *The Halogen Composition of Aerosol Particles over Lake Michigan*, pp. 36–42, *Modern Trends in Activation Analysis*, *Conference Proceedings*. U.S. National Bureau of Standards Special Publication 312.

LUDWIG J. H., MORGAN G. B. and McMULLEN R. B. (1970) Trends in urban air quality. *Trans. Am. geophys. Un.* **51**, 468–475.

PIERRARD J. M. (1969) Photochemical decomposition of lead halides from automobile exhaust. *Environ. Sci. Technol.* **3**, 48–51.

RAY B. J. (1969) M. S. thesis, Department of Chemistry, University of Hawaii.

ROBINSON E. and LUDWIG F. L. (1969) Particle size distribution of urban lead aerosols. *J. Air. Pollut. Control. Ass.* **9**, 664–669.

WINCHESTER J. W., ZOLLER W. H., DUCE R. A. and BENSON C. A. (1967) Lead and halogens in pollution aerosols and snow from Fairbanks. Alaska. *Atmospheric Environment* **1**, 105–119.

15

Airborne Lead and Carbon Monoxide at 45th Street, New York City

JOHN L. BOVÉ
STANLEY SIEBENBERG

The Department of Air Resources of the City of New York has initiated a program to monitor the lead content of the city's air. This effort is part of a larger monitoring program that includes the analyses of 12 metals collected at 38 sampling sites (New York City's Aerometric Network).

This report includes lead concentrations at 6 m above street level at 110 East 45th Street and lead concentrations at two other elevated sampling sites in Manhattan—the Central Park Arsenal Building (Fifth Avenue and 64th Street) and at 240 Second Avenue. The sampling probes at the Central Park Arsenal Building and at 240 Second Avenue were located at an approximate height of 14 and 30 m, respectively. The 45th Street data represent the lead levels collected during a 10-week period from 12 January to 22 March 1969. Additionally, carbon monoxide readings are included for the same 10-week period for the 45th Street site. The lead was monitored by a sequential tape sampler. Two-hour spots were collected at 0.007 m³/min with Whatman No. 4 tape. The carbon monoxide was measured with nondispersive infrared analyzer. The concentrations of lead and carbon monoxide are reported in micrograms per cubic meter and parts per million, respectively.

A previous study (1) at the 45th Street site showed this section of the city to be high in traffic volume and carbon monoxide pollution.

Equipment capable of collecting 2-hour sequential lead samples and continually monitoring for carbon monoxide concentrations was already present at 45th Street as part of a continuing effort by this department. The sampling probe for lead was located at approximately 6 m above street level and 2.6 m in from the curb. The carbon monoxide sampling probe was located approximately 6 m above street level and 3 m in from the curb. Lead samples were collected from the air over 2-hour periods, 24 hours per day, 7 days per week. The carbon monoxide concentrations were continuously monitored, 24 hours per day, 7 days per week. The average 2-hour concentrations of lead and carbon monoxide for the 10-week period between the hours of 8:00 a.m. and 6:00 p.m. were 9.3 $\mu g/m^3$ and 18 ppm, respectively. The carbon monoxide results are compatible with the previously reported results for 45th Street where the earlier investigators reported that the average hourly concentrations exceeded 15 ppm from 9:00 a.m. to 7:00 p.m. The carbon monoxide in both studies exceeded New York State's proposed standards.

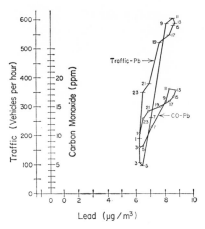

Fig. 2. Lead concentrations, traffic volume and lead concentrations, and carbon monoxide concentration curves at East 45th Street, New York City.

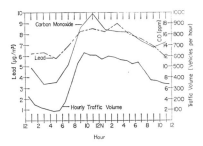

Fig. 1. Two-hour average lead concentrations in grams per cubic meter, carbon monoxide in parts per million, and hourly average traffic in vehicles per hour at East 45th Street, New York City.

The means of the daily averages were 7.5 $\mu g/m^3$ for lead and 13 ppm of carbon monoxide for the 10-week period of the study. Similar results were reported (2) in another New York City study (on Broadway between 34th and 35th Streets). Here the authors reported an annual average for lead of 7.9 $\mu g/m^3$.

The frequency distribution for lead concentrations in the 2-hour samples (812 samples in milligrams per cubic meter), grouped in class intervals of 0 to 4.4, 4.5 to 8.4, 8.5 to 12.4, 12.5 to 16.4, and 16.5 to 20.4, was 32, 35, 16, 9, and 4 percent, respectively. During this same period, eight 2-hour readings were reported between 20.5 and 24.4 $\mu g/m^3$, six between 25.5 and 28.4, two between 28.5 and 32.4, and one greater than 34.

When the lead and carbon monoxide concentrations were plotted against time the curves were similar in shape. These results are shown in Fig. 1. Both pollutants show peak values at 11:00 a.m. and later at 3:00 p.m. Plots of traffic volumes typical of 1967 at 45th Street correlate excellently with the pollutant plots (Fig. 1); this would indicate fixed traffic volume for 45th Street.

We smoothed the curves by calculating moving averages for carbon monoxide, lead concentrations, and traffic volumes. We then plotted the resulting moving averages—lead concentrations* against carbon monoxide concentrations and traffic volumes (eliminating time). The results produced closed curves reminiscent of Lissajous figures (Fig. 2), thereby reinforcing the idea that correlations exist between lead and carbon monoxide and lead and traffic. Two other studies (2, 3) also report correlation between lead and carbon monoxide. The same graph of carbon monoxide plotted against the 1967 traffic count showed that carbon monoxide was a function of traffic (Fig. 3); it can be described by the equation $x = 1.53y^{0.368}$ ($x =$ carbon monoxide in parts per million, and $y =$ traffic in vehicles per hour).

We determined lead concentrations at Central Park (12-m elevation) and 240 Second Avenue (30-m elevation) for a 10-day period during the interval 23 January 1969 through 12 March 1969. The daily average for Central Park for this period was 0.97 μg/m³; for Second. Avenue the concentration for the same period was 1.57 μg/m³. In another recent New York City study (4) the investigation reported annual mean lead concentrations of 3.82 and 2.99 μg/m³ for the Bronx and Manhattan, respectively.

Similar lead concentrations were found at other elevated monitoring sites connected with the Aerometric Network. These lower values at rooftop sites suggest the need for a vertical profile for lead. This work is now in progress, and, in addition, lead concentrations are to be monitored at other sites of high traffic volume in New York.

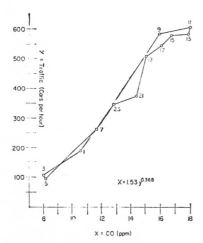

Fig. 3. Carbon monoxide concentration and traffic volume curves at East 45th Street, New York City.

References and Notes

1. K. L. Johnson, L. H. Dworetsky, A. N. Heller, *Science* **160**, 67 (1968).
2. J. M. Collucci, C. R. Begeman, C. R. Kumler, K. Kumler, *J. Air Pollut. Control Ass.* **19**, 4 (1969).
3. Working Group on Lead Contamination, *U.S. Public Health Serv. Publ. 999-AP-12* (U.S. Dept. of Health, Education, and Welfare, Jan. 1965).
4. T. J. Kneip, M. Eisenbud, C. D. Strehlow, P. C. Freudnethal, 62nd annual meeting of the Air Pollution Control Administration, New York City, 22–26 June 1969.

PARTICULATE Pb, ^{210}Pb AND ^{210}Po IN THE ENVIRONMENT*

J. C. LANGFORD

INTRODUCTION

MANY studies[1] have been made of ^{210}Po, ^{210}Pb and stable Pb concentrations in the environment. Polonium-210 and ^{210}Pb are of special interest since both are bone-seeking[2] and are potentially more hazardous[3,4] to the human body than are some other ingested radio-isotopes. Polonium-210 and ^{210}Pb are naturally introduced into the environment by the decay of ^{238}U with a gaseous intermediate, ^{222}Rn $(t_{1/2} = 3.823$ days), which becomes dispersed throughout the atmosphere. Investigations of the ^{210}Pb, Pb and ^{210}Po concentrations in the environs which have been initiated include: stratospheric circulation of ^{210}Po and ^{210}Pb,[5] the measurement of ^{210}Pb in surface air and precipitation,[6] the seasonal variations of ^{210}Pb in ground level air,[7] and the study of lead aerosols in the marine atmosphere.[8] These investigations have shown that the specific activity of ^{210}Pb may become diluted

* This paper is based on work performed under United States Atomic Energy Commission Contract AT(45–1)–1830.

19

in the environs because of the increased concentrations of stable lead pollutants. Since the rapid industrial growth of recent years, stable lead concentrations have increased in the environment.[9]

The accumulation of lead in soils over a period of approximately 40 yr has been compared for areas of high and low motor vehicle traffic densities.[10] When the density was less than 80 vehicles per square mile, no lead accumulations were observed, but where the density was greater than 580 vehicles per square mile, concentrations of lead in the surface 2.5 cm of soil increased by two- to threefold. These increased levels are near industrial areas[11,12] producing certain paint products and in areas having excessive vehicular emissions. Although present levels[13–17] may not be hazardous to the human body, extensive studies are being made to determine the extent of systematic damage to many mammals and the possible synergistic effects in man of ^{210}Po and ^{210}Pb with organic and inorganic aerosols. These investigations are directed toward concentration studies of lead in various organs, blood, and excretion products of the body. Stable lead accumulates[18] with age in the soft tissues of many Americans due to increased exposure to higher atmospheric lead levels in our industrial society. The same accumulation is not observed in countries which have a reduced industrial output.

There have been relatively few studies of stable lead in the marine environment[19] with most oceanic investigations using isolated measurements of stable lead. Systematic measurements[20] of major and minor elements must be made in oceanic areas to permit a more accurate estimate of transport and deposition properties of ocean currents, the elemental distributions in the ocean, rates of vertical mixing in the ocean, and the exchange rates across the air–sea interface. The measurements of particulates Pb, ^{210}Pb and ^{210}Po presented in this paper were made as part of a program designed to characterize the distribution and behavior of radionuclide and trace element concentrations in various oceanic processes.

PROCEDURE

Ocean water was sequentially filtered through 305 mm dia. Millipore filters which removed the >0.3 μ particulate material and through a 0.63 cm thick by 305 mm dia. sorption bed of aluminum oxide which removed soluble material. Particulates in air were removed by filtering air through a similar 230 cm^2 Millipore filter.

A 1 g aliquot of filter paper, associated with lead carrier, and ^{208}Po and ^{212}Pb spikes was dissolved in a mixture of HNO_3 and $HClO_4$ acids. After evaporation to fumes of $HClO_4$, the solution was cooled, diluted to 350 ml with 0.6 M HCl, ascorbic acid was added to reduce ferric iron, and the solution was heated to about 90°C. Polonium-210 was spontaneously deposited on silver discs[21] and analyzed by its alpha emission. The ^{208}Po spike was added to allow a radiochemical yield determination. After careful addition of about 1 ml of concentrated HNO_3 to destroy the excessive ascorbic acid, the solution was evaporated to $HClO_4$ fumes and diluted to 75 ml with 0.6 M HCl. Stable Pb, ^{210}Pb and ^{212}Pb spike[22] were extracted twice with 1% diethylammonium diethlydithiocarbamate (DDTC) and back-extracted twice using 10 ml of 8 M HCl. After evaporating to about 1 ml, the solutions were diluted to about 10 ml, 2 ml of 9 M NaI was added and each sample was extracted twice with 10.0 ml of hexone (prewashed with 1 M HCl). The chemical yield was measured by the analysis of the ^{212}Pb spike. Stable lead was determined in a 2 ml aliquot of the 20 ml organic extract by atomic absorption procedures at 284 nm. The remaining 18 ml were taken to dryness, the organic residue was destroyed by fuming with concentrated HNO_3, and the solution was transferred to a stainless steel planchet. Following the complete decay of the ^{212}Pb spike and complete buildup of the ^{210}Bi daughter of ^{210}Pb, the ^{210}Pb was measured by beta counting the ^{210}Bi daughter through a 6.42 mg/cm^2 aluminum absorber. The analytical precision was determined by using radiochemical spikes.

21

DISCUSSION

Particulate [210]Po, ^{210}Pb and stable Pb concentrations in a Pacific Ocean depth profile are shown in Table 1. The samples were taken at 41°N. Lat., 131°W. Long., which is approximately 350 miles west of the Oregon Coast. The particulate [210]Po and ^{210}Pb concentrations decrease with depth to 656 m, below which they remain fairly constant. These results are in agreement with the [226]Ra measurements made on the same samples,[23] except that the [226]Ra concentrations increased from 656 to 1639 m depths.

The stable lead concentrations also show a decrease with depth to 1639 m. This low value is approaching that reported by TATSUMOTO and PATTERSON[24], who show a nearly constant lead concentration of about 0.02 μg/l. below 2000 m. Lead is present in seawater largely as a particulate. If one assumes that the lead in seawater is primarily from the deposition of airborne aerosols from the industrial consumption of petroleum which began its rapid increase in 1940[25] and that the concentration of lead at 1639 m is due to lead deposited at the surface in 1940,[26] then a good correlation between the concentrations of lead at various depths and the world crude oil production can be made. Thus the large increase of stable lead in the oceans represents atmospheric fallout over a 27 yr period (1940–1967). A least squares fit of the data to the equation $Y = A + BX$ gave $Y = -0.002 + 0.0141\,X$ where $Y = \mu$g Pb/l. and $X =$ billions of barrels of oil. Since this apparent relationship has a standard deviation of 0.020 which includes 0.00, the model was reduced to $Y = 0.014\,X$. This model oversimplifies the actual situation; however, the correlation coefficient of the data is 0.92 indicating a high degree of correlation.

Particulate [210]Po, ^{210}Pb and stable lead concentrations in Atlantic Ocean surface seawater are shown in Table 2. The average concentrations of [210]Po and ^{210}Pb are 0.016 and 0.012 dis/min/l., respectively. In general, the [210]Po concentrations exceed those of [210]Pb. In many lakes and in the Arctic Ocean, the [210]Po/^{210}Pb ratio[27] in fish equals or exceeds 20.

22

Depth (m)†	^{210}Po (dis/min/l)	^{210}Pb (dis/min/l)	Pb (μg/l)	Specific activity ^{210}Pb (dis/min/μg Pb)
20‡	0.14	0.12	2.1	0.057
20	0.049	0.049	0.23	0.21
328	0.031	0.010	0.069	0.14
656	0.014	0.029	0.10	0.29
984	0.024	0.012	0.060	0.20
1639	0.018	0.009	0.036	0.25

* The standard deviation of the combined chemical and radiochemical measurements is ±20%.

† Samples collected at 41°N. Lat. and 131°W. Long.

‡ Sample filter coated with some algae.

The average ratio of ^{210}Po/^{210}Pb in the Pacific Ocean profile was 1.21, which is almost equal to the average in the Atlantic Ocean surface sample of 1.26. A comparison of the oceanic ^{210}Po and ^{210}Pb concentrations with the ^{226}Ra parent shows that they are about tenfold lower than the ^{226}Ra in surface water. This discrepancy may be partially explained by a significant fraction of ^{222}Rn gas escaping to the atmosphere from the mixing layer and the preferential absorption of ^{210}Po and ^{210}Pb compared to ^{226}Ra by marine organisms.[20]

In addition, the particulate lead concentrations in the Atlantic Ocean surface water were measured as a function of distance from the United States (from the eastern coast of Florida). Except for one sample (25° 30'N. Lat., 74°W. Long.), there is a rapid decrease in the particulate lead concentrations to a distance of 1440 miles. Thereafter, the concentrations slowly decrease by approximately 20% to near the African coast. It seems that the source of particulate lead in the ocean is primarily of terrestrial origin, presumably by air pollution since the physical barriers of the Bahama Islands and the Gulf Stream would prevent most eastward flows of mainland rivers from the Florida coast. The specific activity of ^{210}Pb in the Pacific Ocean depth profile averaged 0.191 dis/min/μg Pb and varied from

Table 2. Pb, ^{210}Pb and ^{210}Po concentrations in surface Atlantic Ocean water

| Location | | ^{210}Po | ^{210}Pb | Pb | Specific activity ^{210}Pb | Distance from U.S.A. |
N. Lat	W. Long	(dis/min/l)	(dis/min/l)	(μg/l)	(dis/min/μg Pb)	statute miles
25°30'	74°	0.007 ± 0.007	0.009 ± 0.002	0.45 ± 0.04	0.020	480
25°33'	72°20'	0.015 ± 0.001	0.016 ± 0.002	2.23 ± 0.02	0.0072	600
25°10'	65°55'	0.014 ± 0.001	0.015 ± 0.002	0.72 ± 0.05	0.021	1030
24°28'	62°18'	0.018 ± 0.002	0.011 ± 0.002	0.31 ± 0.03	0.036	1320
24°48'	59°20'	0.017 ± 0.001	0.012 ± 0.002	0.25 ± 0.03	0.048	1440
8°50'	38°28'	0.022 ± 0.002	0.008 ± 0.002	0.24 ± 0.03	0.030	3000
5°48'	16°35'	0.017 ± 0.002	0.017 ± 0.002	0.21 ± 0.03	0.081	4570

0.057 to 0.29 dis/min/μg Pb. These values are considerably higher than the average specific activity in the samples from the Atlantic Ocean surface profile. The ^{210}Pb varied from 0.007 dis/min/μg Pb in the sample at 25° 30′N Lat., to 0.081 dis/min/μg Pb in the sample collected at 5°48′N. Lat., with an overall average of 0.035 dis/min/μg Pb over the 4000 mile profile distance.

The observed data suggest that washout and gravitational settling have removed most of the particulate lead particles large enough to be affected by these processes by a distance of 1440 miles. After 1440 miles, the slowly decreasing concentrations of particulate lead suggest a nearly constant input of lead into this part of the ocean. The low concentration of particulate lead in the sample at 1440 miles from the United States is probably due to the prevailing wind and oceanic circulation in the area. The Gulf Stream[29,30] brings in water from the south and the east, where the possibility of industrial pollution is greatly reduced. The input of stable particulate lead into the oceans at 0–25°N. Lat., is derived from inter-mixing across the Subtropical High Pressure Belt at 35°N. Lat. Since it has been postulated that the sources of lead are of industrial and vehicular origin, then the output would also be related to the output of CO_2. The computed maximum of the distribution[31] for industrial CO_2 output occurs at 45°N. Lat., and nearly 90% of the total output appears between 30°N. Lat., to 60°N. Lat.

Table 3 gives representative data of world-wide measurements of ^{210}Pb and stable lead in air and water for comparison to the marine environment. Although there are large variations in concentration between different sources, the urban-industrial concentrations of stable lead in air are much higher than other airborne sources. These differences in concentration[32] reflect local conditions, distances from industrial sources. These differences in concentration[32] reflect local conditions, distances from industrial sources, and the concentration of traffic and internal combustion engines. The concentration of stable lead in rainwater should vary as

Table 3. *Concentrations of ^{210}Po, ^{210}Pb and stable Pb in air and water in the environs*

Air

	^{210}Pb (dis/min/m³)	Pb (µg/m³)
Urban		0.82 (avg)[9] 0.1–3.2 (range)[9]
Rural	0.006 ± 0.0001† 0.02–0.11 (range)[1]	0.00035 ± 0.00003† 0.05[33]
Marine		0.0003–0.0015[8,]

Water

	^{210}Po (dis/min/l.)	^{210}Pb (dis/min/l.)	Pb (µg/L.)
Rain		4.0 (mean)[34] 2.2–22 (range)[1]	17.4 (mean)[34]
Inland surface		0.19–15 (range)[1]	
Marine	0.030 ± 0.004*	0.024 ± 0.005*	0.22 ± 0.04‡

* Average values from Tables 1 and 2.
† Determined in a desert area of the State of Washington (Hanford area).
‡ Best estimate of ocean surface background concentration.

its proximity to the source of lead pollution. Several studies of inland waters[1,27] indicate that ^{210}Pb is rapidly removed from the surface water, which suggests that stable lead may also be scavenged. However, the mechanisms for removal of stable lead in the ocean apparently are much different than in lakes since depth profiles of particulate lead in the ocean show lower concentrations at great depths relative to the surface. The transport of particulate Pb in seawater is complicated especially through the turbulent mixing layer to the thermocline. In this paper the effect of the mixing layer which undoubtedly is responsible for the low particulate Pb concentration at the 328 m depth has been ignored. A more complete mathematical description of the rate of transfer of material through this layer along with long term "average" layer thickness and the subsequent settling process is required to determine transport processes in the ocean.

REFERENCES

1. Z. JAWOROSKI, Radioactive lead in the environment and in the human body, *G.E.C. atom. Energy Rev.* **7**, 3 (1969).
2. I.C.R.P. Recommendations: Report 2, *Permissible Dose of Internal Radiation*. Pergamon Press, New York (1960).
3. A. V. ASTIN, N.C.R.P. Rep. No. 30, U.S. Dept. of Commerce, *Safe Handling of Radioactive Materials*, 9 March (1964).
4. I.C.R.P. Report 11, *A Review of the Radiosensitivity of Tissues in Bone*, Pergamon Press, New York (1968).
5. A. C. STERN, *Air-Polution*, Vol. 1, 2nd Edition. Academic Press, New York (1968).
6. L. U. JOSHI, C. RANGARAJAN and SARADA GOPALAKRISHNAN, Measurement of lead-210 in surface air and precipitation. *Tellus* **21**, 107 (1969).
7. L. U. JOSHI and T. N. MAHADEVAN, Seasonal variations of radium-D (lead-210) in ground level air in India, *Health Phys.* **15**, 67 (1968).
8. T. J. CHOW, J. L. EARL and C. F. BENNETT, Lead aerosols in marine atmosphere, *Envir. Sci. Tech.* **3**, 737 (1969).
9. C. D. BURNHAM, C. E. MOORE and E. KANABROCKI, Determination of lead in airborne particulates in Chicago and Cook County, Ill. by atomic absorption, *Envir. Sci. Tech.* **3**, 472

(1969).

10. A. L. PAGE and T. J. GANJE, Accumulation of lead in soils for regions of high and low motor vehicle density, *Envir. Sci. Tech.* **4,** 140 (1970).

11. T. J. CHOW and M. S. JOHNSTONE, Lead isotopes in gasoline and aerosols of Los Angeles basin, Calif. *Science* **147,** 502 (1965).

12. A. L. LAZRUS, E. LORANGE and J. P. LODGE, JR., Lead and other metal ions in U.S. precipitation, *Envir. Sci. Tech.* **4,** 55 (1970).

13. R. B. HOLTZMAN, Measurement of the natural contents of RaD (^{210}Pb) and RaF (^{210}Po) in human bone-estimates of whole body burdens, *Health Phys.* **9,** 385 (1963).

14. R. L. BLANCHARD, Concentrations of ^{210}Pb and ^{210}Po in human soft tissues, *Health Phys.* **13,** 625 (1967).

15. E. J. BARATTA, J. C. APIDIANAKIS and E. S. FERRI, Cesium-137, lead-210 and polonium-210 concentrations in selected human tissues in the U.S., *Am. ind. Hyg. Ass. J.* **30,** 443 (1969).

16. N. COHEN and G. P. HOWELLS, A brief review of ^{210}Pb metabolism, *Fallout Program Q. Summary Report*, HASL-204, pp. 81–97 (1969).

17. L. J. GOLDWATER and A. W. HOOVER, An international study of "normal" levels of lead in blood and urine, *Arch. Envir. Health* **15,** p. 60 (1967).

18. H. A. SCHROEDER and I. H. TIPTON, The human body burden of lead, *Arch. Envir. Health* **17,** 965 (1968).

19. V. G. KORT, *Chemistry of the Pacific Oceans*, Vol. 3, pp. 297. Inst. of Oceanogr., U.S.S.R., Acad. of Sci. (1966).

20. D. E. ROBERTSON, L. A. RANCITELLI and R. W. PERKINS, Multielement analysis of seawater, marine organisms, and sediments by neutron activation without chemical separations. Presented at the *Int. Symp. Applic. Neutron Activation Anal. Oceanogr.*, Brussels, Belgium, June, pp. 17–22 (1968).

21. S. C. BLACK, Low level polonium and radiolead analysis, *Health Phys.* **7,** 87 (1961).

22. J. C. LANGFORD, Procedure for the determination of lead-210 and total lead in biological samples, *Anal. Chem.* **41,** 1716 (1969).

23. D. E. ROBERTSON, W. O. FORSTER, H. G. RIECK and J. C. LANGFORD, A study of the trace element and radionuclide behavior in a northeast Pacific Ocean ecosystem 350 miles off Newport, Oregon, *Pacif. Northwest Lab. Annual Rep. for 1967, Vol. II: Phys. Sci.* , Part 2, *Radiological Sci.* BNWL-715, Part 2, pp. 92–108. Pacif. Northwest Lab., Richland, Wash. (1968).

24. M. Tatsumoto and C. C. Patterson, Concentrations of common lead in some Atlantic and Mediterranean waters and in snow, *Nature, Lond.* **199,** 350 (1963).

25. U.S. Bureau of Census, 88th Ed., p. 694 (World production of crude petroleum) (1967).

26. M. G. Gross, Sinking rates of radioactive fallout particles in the northeast Pacif. Ocean, 1961–62, *Nature Lond.* **216,** 670 (1967).

27. P. Kauranen, ^{210}Po and ^{210}Pb concentrations of some water and fish samples from Finland. Presented at the 5th *R.I.S. Symp.*, Helsinki, Finland, May, pp. 19–20 (1969).

28. T. M. Beasley, Lead-210 in selected marine organisms. Thesis, Oregon State University (1969).

29. J. P. Riley and G. Skirrow, *Chemical Oceanography,* Vol. 1, pp. 44–47. Academic Press, New York (1965).

30. K. Yoshida, *Studies on Oceanography,* pp. 55–58. University of Washington Press, Seattle (1965).

31. B. Bolin and C. D. Keeling, Large-scale atmospheric mixing as deduced from seasonal and meridional variations of carbon dioxide, *J. geophys. Res.* **68,** 3899 (1963).

32. M. Neiburger, What factors determine the optimum size area for an air pollution control program. *Proc. 3rd Nat. Conf. Air Pollution,* Wash., D.C., pp. 442–449, 12–13 December (1966). U.S. Dept. of Health, Education and Welfare, Public Health Service (1967).

33. C. C. Patterson, Contaminated and natural lead environments of man, *Arch. Envir. Health* **11,** 344 (1965).

34. G. L. Ter Haar, R. B. Holtzman and H. F. Lucas, Jr., Lead and lead-210 in rainwater, *Nature, Lond.* **216,** No. 5113, 353 (1967).

Lead In The Environment:
Soil, Plants, Water, Diet

DIETARY INTAKE OF ^{210}Pb

ROBERT S. MORSE and GEORGE A. WELFORD

INTRODUCTION

THE ASSESSMENT of ^{210}Pb in the human body is important because of the biological effect of its daughter activity, ^{210}Po. It has been reported that the radiation exposure to the body from ^{210}Po is greater than the exposure from Ra^{226} and ^{90}Sr.[1,2] This is particularly true for some northern diets.[3,4]

This study presents data on the ^{210}Pb content of normal diets for New York City, as based on the selected food consumption figures of the U.S. Department of Agriculture.[5] Only ^{210}Pb (and not ^{210}Po) was measured in all samples analyzed because the ^{210}Po/^{210}Pb ratio for diet samples is usually unity.[6,7] Stable lead and ^{226}Ra values are also given for the New York City diet to check whether there is any correlation between ^{210}Pb, ^{226}Ra and stable lead.

ANALYTICAL METHOD

The method used for ^{210}Pb analyses was similar to that described by PETROW.[8] Samples were prepared by wet ashing in the presence of lead carrier, using nitric acid so that no lead would be volatilized. Recoveries of the carrier were determined by atomic absorption measurement. Bismuth-210 was separated from the ^{210}Pb as bismuth oxychloride after equilibration. This precipitate was covered with aluminum foil (7.2 mg/cm^2) to absorb alpha particles from any ^{210}Po that was not completely removed and the ^{210}Bi determined by beta scintillation counting. Reagent blanks were run periodically and purity of the ^{210}Bi was measured, when possible, by measuring the half-life of the beta activity.

The entire method was tested using spiked samples as well as samples where ^{210}Pb had already been determined by other procedures.

RESULTS AND DISCUSSION

The amount of ^{210}Pb was measured in 19 categories of food in the New York City diet. These values, as well as stable lead and ^{226}Ra values, are given in Table 1. Stable lead was determined on aliquots of the same samples. Radium-226 was measured in a previous study,[9] but is generally consistent from diet to diet.

The contribution of various food types to the total intake depends on both the concentration and the amount consumed. For example, although shell fish have the highest ^{210}Pb content, their contribution to the intake of ^{210}Pb is low because of the small amount of this food consumed. The ^{210}Pb content of potatoes and bakery products is relatively high, and since the consumption of these items is high the ^{210}Pb intake from them is high. The annual consumption of milk is 200 kg, and though the ^{210}Pb content of milk is low the contribution to intake is high.

The concentration of ^{210}Pb in the New York City diet may be calculated in other units as 0.70 pCi ^{210}Pb/kg food, which is very similar to other diets measured in the United States[10] as shown in Table 2.

Category	kg/yr	^{210}Pb pCi/kg	^{210}Pb pCi/yr	Stable Pb mg/kg	Stable Pb mg/yr	^{226}Ra pCi/kg	^{226}Ra pCi/yr
Fresh fruit	8.0	0.39	3.1	0.049	0.39	0.67	5.4
Shell fish	1.0	3.4	3.4	—	—	0.80	0.80
Poultry	20	0.45	9.0	0.042	0.84	0.76	15
Meat	79	0.49	39	0.060	4.7	0.01	0.79
Eggs	15	0.26	3.9	0.045	0.68	6.1	91
Fresh fruit	59	0.40	24	0.063	3.7	0.43	25
Canned fruit	11	2.0	22	0.17	1.9	0.17	1.9
Fresh vegetables	48	1.1	52	0.059	2.8	0.50	24
Canned vegetables	22	0.44	9.7	0.033	0.73	0.65	14
Root vegetables	10	0.21	2.1	0.039	0.39	1.4	14
Potatoes	38	1.5	57	0.089	3.4	2.8	110
Macaroni	3.0	0.92	2.8	0	0	2.1	6.3
Rice	3.0	0.88	2.6	0.020	0.060	0.76	2.3
Juices	28	0.23	6.4	—	—	0.42	12
Dry beans	3.0	0.76	2.3	0.049	0.15	1.1	3.3
Flour	34	1.3	44	0.022	0.75	1.9	65
Bakery products	44	1.8	78	—	—	2.8	123
Whole grain products	11	2.2	24	0.050	0.55	2.2	24
Milk	200	0.29	58	0.016	3.2	0.25	50
* Yearly intake		440 pCi		24 mg		490 pCi	
* Daily intake		1.2 pCi		0.066 mg		1.6 pCi	
Drinking water							
† Yearly intake (400 kg)		16 pCi					
Daily intake		0.05 pCi					

* See Ref. 5.
† See Ref. 11.

Table 2. *Mean concentrations of* ^{210}Pb *in total diets*

Location	pCi ^{210}Pb/kg	Reference
New York City	0.70 ± 0.04	This paper
Boston	0.82 ± 0.21	
Chicago	0.86 ± 0.21	
New Orleans	0.86 ± 0.10	(10)
Los Angeles	0.69 ± 0.08	
Palmer (Alaska)	0.79 ± 0.09	
Honolulu (Hawaii)	0.75 ± 0.21	
Holtzman (Calculated for USA)	1.0	(12)

Table 3. *Main sources of* ^{210}Pb *in the human body—New York City*

	Daily intake (pCi)	Fraction reaching the blood	Amount of ^{210}Pb reaching the blood (pCi/day)
Air	0.30*	0.29	0.10
Drinking water	0.05	0.08	0.004
Food	1.2	0.08	0.10
Total intake	1.57	0.094	0.21

* Assume 20 m³ of air inhaled daily,[13] and an average concentration as measured of 0.014 pCi/m³ in New York.

The amount of ^{210}Pb reaching the blood can be estimated for food using the ICRP value for the fraction of lead absorbed.[11] This calculation is shown in Table 3, where 1.2 pCi of ^{210}Pb/day in the diet results in 0.1 pCi/day in blood. Air also contributes 0.1

pCi ^{210}Pb to the blood per day and in New York City accounts for approximately 50% of the ^{210}Pb intake as calculated in Table 3.

The stable lead content of New York City foods is also presented in Table 1. There seems

Table 4. Specific activity of ^{210}Pb in New York City foods

Type	pCi ^{210}Pb/kg	mg Pb/kg	pCi ^{210}Pb/g Pb
Fresh fish	0.39	0.049	8000
Poultry	0.45	0.042	10,700
Meat	0.49	0.060	8200
Eggs	0.26	0.045	5800
Root vegetables	0.21	0.039	5400
Rice	0.88	0.020	44,000
Whole grain products	2.22	0.050	44,000
Flour	1.3	0.022	59,000

to be no correlation between ^{210}Pb and stable lead. The specific activities of lead for each food type are shown in Table 4. These values have a range of more than a factor of 10, and would seem to indicate different sources for the ^{210}Pb and stable lead.

Table 1 also seems to indicate no correlation between the amounts of ^{226}Ra and ^{210}Pb in food. Radioactive equilibrium is not to be expected because of the gaseous daughter product of radium, ^{222}Rn, which readily escapes from food.

CONCLUSION

Generally, the overall intake of ^{210}Pb for New York City is similar to ^{210}Pb intake in the United States at various locations. It can be expected that the exposure from ^{210}Pb would not vary much in the United States except where personnel are exposed occupationally to ^{210}Pb.

REFERENCES

1. W. STAHLHOFEN, Assessment of radioactivity in man, IAEA Vienna, Report, p. 505 (1964).
2. J. N. STANNARD and G. W. CASARETT, Radiat. Res. Suppl. 5, 398 (1964).
3. P. KAURANEN and J. K. MIETTINEN, Health Phys. 16, 287 (1969).
4. R. L. BLANCHARD and J. B. MOORE, Health Phys. 18, 127 (1970).
5. US AEC, Health and Safety Lab., Environmental Studies Div., New York, N.Y., Food Purchase Plan.
6. B. GLOBEL, Physicist Thesis Institut for Biophysiks der Universitat des Sarrlandes, Saarbrücken (1966).
7. C. R. HILL, Health Phys. 8, 17 (1962).
8. H. G. PETROW and A. COVER, Analyt. Chem. 37, 13 (1965).
9. Fallout Quarterly Summary Report, USAEC, HASL-224 April (1970).
10. P. J. MAGNO, P. R. GROULX and J. C. APIDIANAKIS, Health Phys. 16, 286 (1970).
11. ICRP, Report of Committee II, p. 217, Pergamon Press, London (1959).
12. R. B. HOLTZMAN, Health Phys. 9, 385 (1963).
13. ICRP, Report of Committee II, p. 152, Pergamon Press, London (1959).

LEAD-210 IN AIR AND TOTAL DIETS IN THE UNITED STATES DURING 1966

P. J. MAGNO, P. R. GROULX and J. C. APIDIANAKIS

INTRODUCTION

RADIATION exposure to man from naturally occuring radionuclides in his environment has been the subject of extensive study in recent years.[1] Many of these studies have been concerned with lead-210 and it has been shown that this radionuclide with its daughter polonium-210 contributes a significant portion of the natural radiation dose to the skeleton.[2,3] It has also been shown that lead-210 is subject to ecological concentration processes in the arctic region[4–8] and is inhaled in cigarette smoke.[9] Numerous measurements of the concentrations of lead-210 in man and his environment have been reported. No data, however, have been reported on measurements of lead-210 in total diets. HOLTZMAN[2] and HILL[4] found it necessary to use excretion measurements to estimate lead-210 intakes. This report presents data on the concentrations of lead-210 in air and diet and discusses geographical variations in these concentrations in the United States. It also compares the various routes of intake of this radionuclide and estimates the relative contributions to the body tissues from the various sources of exposure.

SAMPLE COLLECTION

Air particulates

A portion of a sample of air particulates representing approximately 200–1000 m³ of air was obtained daily during 1966 from selected sampling stations in the Public Health Service's Radiation Alert Network (RAN).[10] Under this program, airborne particulate samples are collected by drawing air through 4-in. MSA No. 2133 "All Dust" filters at high velocity using either a Staplex "Hi Volume" sampler or one of several lobar-type positive displacement air pumps. The samples from each station were composited on a monthly basis. Samples were obtained from the following stations: Anchorage, Alaska; San Juan, Puerto Rico; Honolulu, Hawaii; Winchester, Massachusetts; Salt Lake City, Utah; Springfield, Illinois; New Orleans, Louisiana and Los Angeles, California.

Total diet

Total diet samples were obtained monthly during 1966 from selected stations in the Public Health Service's Institutional Total Diet Sampling Network.[11] These samples represented the

Also to be considered in comparing the data from these locations is the difference in the latitude of the sampling locations. PATTERSON and LOCKHART[16] showed a variation in the lead-210 concentration in air with latitude at the 80th meridian (west). Maximum concentrations were reported at a latitude of about 40° (north) which is the approximate latitude of Springfield, Illinois, and Salt Lake City, Utah.

The mean concentrations of lead-210 in air particulates at Winchester, Massachusetts, and Los Angeles, California, both coastal locations, were a factor of almost two less than the mean concentrations at Springfield, Illinois or Salt Lake City, Utah. It would appear that locations affected by air masses which have passed over ocean waters (and hence lower in radon-222) will have lower lead-210 concentrations than inland locations where the air masses have passed over land areas.

Total diet

The mean concentrations of lead-210 in total diet samples collected from various locations in the United States during 1966 are presented in Table 2 in pCi/kg of food. These mean con-

Table 2. Mean concentrations of lead-210 in total diets during 1966

Location	^{210}Pb (pCi/kg)
Boston, Massachusetts	0.82 ± 0.21
Chicago, Illinois	0.86 ± 0.21
New Orleans, Louisiana	0.86 ± 0.10
Los Angeles, California	0.69 ± 0.08
Palmer, Alaska	0.79 ± 0.09
Honolulu, Hawaii	0.75 ± 0.21

Note: Errors are one standard error of the mean.

centrations ranged from 0.69–0.86 pCi/kg of food. A *t*-test showed that any differences in the mean concentration between locations were not statistically significant ($P = 0.05$). Measurements of lead-210 in water samples obtained for the Institutional Total Diet Sampling Network[11] showed lead-210 concentrations of about 5 fCi/l. It can be concluded from these data that drinking water does not contribute significantly to the dietary intake of lead-210. The mean value for all composite diet samples analyzed was 0.80 pCi/kg and this value would appear to be the best estimate of the lead-210 concentration in diet samples for this age group in the United States. It is surprising that the lead-210 concentrations in total diets from Honolulu, Hawaii were not substantially lower than those at Chicago, Illinois despite the difference of five which occurred in the concentrations of lead-210 in air particulates between these locations.

DISCUSSION

One of the objectives of this study was to establish the relative exposure to standard man from the various environmental sources of lead-210. The samples analyzed during this study were collected as part of the Bureau of Radiological Health's Radiation Alert Network and Institutional Total Diet Sampling Network for the specific objectives of those networks. The following observations, therefore, are limited to the extent that the samples analyzed were not collected for the specific objectives of this study and as a result, certain assumptions and extrapolations have been necessary in interpreting these data for standard man.

Using the data from Tables 1 and 2, and the ICRP models,[17,18] the relative contributions of lead-210 to body tissues of standard man from ingestion and inhalation were estimated from the following formulae.

(1) $A_1 = I_1 f_1$.

A_1 = pCi/day absorbed into the blood stream from ingestion.

I_1 = pCi/day ingested.

f_1 = fraction of ingested lead-210 reaching the blood stream.

(2) $A_2 = I_2 D_5 f_2 + I_2 D_5 f_1 f_3$

A_2 = pCi/day absorbed into blood stream from inhalation.

I_2 = pCi/day inhaled.

D_5 = fraction of inhaled dust deposited in pulmonary compartment.

f_1 = fraction of ingested lead-210 reaching the blood stream.

f_2 = fraction of pulmonary deposited dust absorbed into blood stream.

f_3 = fraction of pulmonary deposited dust transferred to GI tract.

Table 3. *Estimated amounts of lead-210 reaching blood stream from inhalation of air particulates*

Location	^{210}Pb(pCi/day)	% of Intake
Winchester, Massachusetts	0.035	20
Springfield, Illinois	0.066	32
New Orleans, Louisiana	0.053	27
Los Angeles, California	0.038	21
Anchorage, Alaska	0.023	14
Honolulu, Hawaii	0.013	8

The following values were used in these calculations: $f_1 = 0.08$, $f_2 = 0.20$, $f_3 = 0.80$, $D_5 = 0.48$, inhalation rate $= 20$ m³/day, dietary intake $= 2.1$ kg/day.[19] The lead-210 was assumed to be present in a form falling into Class W and to be associated with particles having a mean diameter of 0.13 μ as reported by SHLEIEN.[20] The amounts of lead-210 absorbed into the blood stream from dust particles deposited in the naso-pharyngeal and tracheobronchial compartments are negligible and were not considered in these calculations.

The amount of lead-210 calculated to reach the blood stream from ingestion was 0.14 pCi/day and as indicated previously this value is representative of all the locations sampled. The amounts of lead-210 calculated to reach the blood stream from inhalation varied with location and these values are presented in Table 3.

From these above data it is estimated that an average of 0.15 to 0.21 pCi/day of lead-210 reaches the blood stream of inhabitants of the United States from these sources of exposure and that about 70–90% of this amount comes from ingestion.

Another major source of exposure to lead-210 is the inhalation of this radionuclide in tobacco smoke. FERRI[9] reported an intake of 0.8 pCi of lead-210 from smoking one pack of cigarettes. Particle sizes in tobacco smoke are reported to range from 0.01 to 0.25 micron.[21] No information is presently available on the sizes of the particles with which the lead-210 is associated. If for comparison purposes, it is assumed that the lead-210 in tobacco smoke is associated with particles having a mean diameter similar to that of the lead-210 in air particulates, then the amount of lead-210 reaching the blood stream from smoking one pack of cigarettes per day would be about 0.1 pCi/day. This amount of lead-210 is almost equal to that amount reaching the blood stream from ingestion and would increase the concentrations of lead-210 in body tissues by a factor of 1.5–2.0 depending upon the location. These data would seem to be in agreement with HOLTZMAN[22] who showed that the concentration of lead-210 in bones from smokers was twice that of non-smokers.

REFERENCES

1. J. A. S. ADAMS and W. M. LOWDER, *The Natural Radiation Environment*. University of Chicago Press, Chicago (1964).
2. R. B. HOLTZMAN, *Health Phys.* **9**, 385 (1963).
3. W. STAHLHOFEN, *Assessment of Radioactivity in Man*, Vol. 2, p. 505. IAEA, Vienna (1964).
4. C. R. HILL, *Radiological Concentration Processes*, p. 297. Pergamon Press, Oxford (1967).
5. R. L. BLANCHARD, *Radiological Concentration Processes*, p. 281. Pergamon Press, Oxford (1967).
6. R. B. HOLTZMAN, *The Pb-210 (RaD) Concentrations of Some Biological Materials from Arctic Regions*. ANL-6769, 59 (1963).
7. T. M. BEASLEY and H. E. PALMER, *Science* **152**, 1062 (1966).
8. R. L. BLANCHARD and J. W. KEARNEY, *Environ. Sci. Technol.* **1**, 932 (1967).
9. E. S. FERRI and H. CHRISTIANSEN, *Publ. Hlth Rept.* **82**, 828 (1967).
10. Public Health Service, *Radiol. Hlth Data* **7**, 658 (1966).
11. Public Health Service, *Radiol. Hlth Data* **8**, 591 (1967).
12. D. H. PEIRSON, R. S. CAMBRAY and G. S. SPICER, *Tellus* **18**, 427 (1965).
13. L. U. JOSHI and T. N. MAHADEVAN, *Health Phys.* **15**, 67 (1968).

14. F. Barreria, *Science* **190,** 1092 (1961).
15. R. B. Holtzman, *Health Phys.* **11,** 477 (1965).
16. R. L. Patterson and L. B. Lockhart, *The Natural Radiation Environment*, p. 383. University of Chicago Press, Chicago (1964).
17. *ICRP Publication* 2. Pergamon Press, Oxford (1959).
18. Task Group on Lung Dynamics, *Health Phys.* **12,** 173 (1966).
19. State of California Department of Public Health, Bureau of Radiological Health, *Radiol. Hlth. Data* **9,** 261 (1968).
20. B. Shleien, A. G. Friend and H. A. Thomas, Jr., *Health Phys.* **13,** 513 (1967).
21. T. F. Hatch and P. Gross, *Pulmonary Deposition and Retention of Inhaled Aerosols*. Academic Press, New York (1964).
22. R. B. Holtzman and F. H. Ilcewicz, *Science* **153,** 1259 (1966).

^{210}Pb AND ^{210}Po IN TISSUES OF SOME ALASKAN RESIDENTS AS RELATED TO CONSUMPTION OF CARIBOU OR REINDEER MEAT

R. L. BLANCHARD and J. B. MOORE

INTRODUCTION

ELEVATED levels of the fission products ^{90}Sr and ^{137}Cs exist in certain Alaskan populations that include caribou meat as a portion of their diet.[1-5] These radionuclides enter the arctic ecosystem as fallout from nuclear detonations and are accumulated by lichens which are consumed in large quantities by caribou and reindeer.[2,4] In addition to ^{90}Sr and ^{137}Cs, ^{210}Pb and ^{210}Po have also been observed to be in high concentrations in lichens and in bones and some soft tissues of caribou, while in the muscle of the latter, high levels of ^{210}Po have been observed.[6-9] For this reason, it has been suggested that populations who consume a regular diet of caribou or reindeer meat may also have high body burdens of ^{210}Pb and ^{210}Po. The latter, being an alpha emitter, is particularly hazardous in high concentrations with respect to internal radiation exposure.[10]

The body burden of ^{137}Cs has been measured extensively throughout the caribou eating populations of Alaksa by whole-body counting techniques employing gamma-spectrometry.[3-5,11]

The measurement of the body burden of ^{210}Pb and ^{210}Po in this population, however, is considerably more difficult. Measurements must be conducted on autopsy tissue by radiochemical techniques. The difficult task of obtaining appropriate specimens is reflected in the scarcity of reported measurements. HILL has reported the ^{210}Po concentrations in 18 samples of human placenta,[12] and the ^{210}Pb content of 3 bone samples from northern Canada.[8] In addition, HOLTZMAN has reported concentrations of ^{210}Pb and ^{210}Po in 3 placenta and 1 blood sample from subjects residing near Barrow, Alaska.[7]

As a result of the absence of ^{210}Po and ^{210}Pb measurements in tissues from the Alaskan Eskimo, it has been possible only to compute an approximate body burden of these nuclides from either the analyses of caribou meat with an estimated intake or from urine analyses. From the latter, BEASLEY and PALMER have estimated that the average ^{210}Po body burden of people living at Anaktuvuk Pass, Alaska is 3.5 nCi.[9]

It has been generally accepted that the source of the ^{210}Pb in the arctic ecosystem, as in other regions, is from the decay of atmospheric ^{222}Rn.[6-9] Lead atoms so formed return to the earth's surface primarily in rainfall and are continually accumulated by the slow growing, long living arctic lichen. During this time, ^{210}Po grows into near radioactive equilibrium with the ^{210}Pb. It has been suggested, however, that a major fraction of the ^{210}Pb deposited in recent years was produced in atmospheric nuclear detonations by the reaction ^{208}Pb$(2n,\gamma)$ ^{210}Pb.[14]

The purpose of this study was to investigate the increased tissue levels of ^{210}Pb and ^{210}Po associated with the consumption of caribou meat. In addition, to ascertain the significance of atmospheric nuclear detonations as a source of ^{210}Pb in the arctic, the concentration of ^{210}Pb in recently collected lichen and caribou bone was compared with the concentration in similar samples collected before 1951. Radium-226 was also measured in these older samples so that the ^{210}Pb concentrations could be corrected for ingrowth.

EXPERIMENTAL

The analytical procedure employed for the determination of ^{210}Pb and ^{210}Po has been described previously.[15,16] The samples were wet ashed in nitric acid and 72 % perchloric acid and the ^{210}Po was deposited on a 2-in. silver disc from a 0.5 N HCl solution containing 200 mg of ascorbic acid at 85°C. The ^{210}Pb present was calculated from the ^{210}Po ingrowth, which was measured by repeating the ^{210}Po deposition on another silver disc 3–4 months after the initial deposition. The alpha activity of the ^{210}Po deposited on the disc was measured in a low-background (0.5–0.8 counts/hr) ZnS(Ag) scintillation counter. The initial ^{210}Po values obtained were corrected for decay and ingrowth from the ^{210}Pb to obtain the concentration at the time of death.

Any muscle attached to the bone was removed and the bones were fat extracted in anhydrous benzene. Defatting the bones was performed in order to give a more reproducible bone sample weight,[17] and it was determined that neither ^{210}Pb nor ^{210}Po was removed during the extraction. The average ratio of defat weight/fresh weight was 0.46 ± 0.08 (S.D.) for 30 rib samples.

The ^{226}Ra content was measured by the radon emanation method.[18,19] In each case, the ^{226}Ra content was measured in the same sample used for the ^{210}Pb analysis.

RESULTS AND DISCUSSION

Human tissues

In Table 1 are listed the data for the Alaskan subjects from which tissue samples were obtained for analysis. The subjects are listed in the order of increasing caribou consumption, and the table includes the age, sex, residence and a brief statement on the frequency with which caribou was eaten. Although it would be more desirable to have knowledge of exact quantities of caribou or reindeer consumed, such data was not available.

Listed in Table 2 are the concentrations of ^{210}Po and ^{210}Pb measured in the various tissues.

Table 1. Human sample data

Subject number	Age	Sex	Alaskan residence	Caribou in diet
1	6	F	Platinum	None
2	15	M	Anchorage	None
3	40	F	Point Barrow and Anchorage	Ate caribou meat regularly at Barrow, but had lived in Anchorage the last three years where she ate none
4	78	M	Eagle	Ate caribou meat occasionally
5	65	M	Akiak (near Bethel)	A few times a year
6	25	F	Anchorage	Ate caribou meat once or twice a month
7	55	M	Kivalina	Caribou meat was main diet in winter—fish in summer
8	77	M	Koyuk	A steady diet of reindeer meat, but ate none during terminal illness of 3 months

Table 2. *Concentrations of* ^{210}Po *and* ^{210}Pb *in human tissues from Alaska*

Subject	^{210}Po (pCi/kg)	^{210}Pb (pCi/kg)	^{210}Po/^{210}Pb	Subject	^{210}Po (pCi/kg)	^{210}Pb (pCi/kg)	^{210}Po/^{210}Pb
	Lung				Muscle		
1	0.9 ± 0.1	1.2 ± 0.1	0.8 ± 0.1	1	3.0 ± 0.4	2.1 ± 0.4	1.4 ± 0.3
2	4.5 ± 0.3	5.1 ± 0.4	0.9 ± 0.1	2	1.8 ± 0.2	1.5 ± 0.3	1.2 ± 0.3
4	2.8 ± 0.2	3.5 ± 0.4	0.8 ± 0.1	3	1.1 ± 0.3	1.3 ± 0.3	0.9 ± 0.2
5	3.5 ± 0.2	3.8 ± 0.4	0.9 ± 0.1	4	3.3 ± 0.5	1.7 ± 0.3	1.9 ± 0.4
6	22 ± 1	7.0 ± 0.7	3.1 ± 0.3	5	1.2 ± 0.2	3.4 ± 0.5	0.35 ± 0.07
8	25 ± 1	10.3 ± 0.7	2.4 ± 0.2	7	6.1 ± 0.3	2.2 ± 0.3	2.8 ± 0.4
				8	10.6 ± 0.7	5.0 ± 0.4	2.1 ± 0.2
	Liver				Spleen		
1	12.1 ± 0.5	9.8 ± 0.8	1.2 ± 0.1	1	1.3 ± 0.2	1.1 ± 0.2	1.2 ± 0.2
2	13.6 ± 0.4	15 ± 0.1	0.92 ± 0.04	2	3.9 ± 0.2	4.2 ± 0.3	0.93 ± 0.08
3	11.7 ± 0.7	4.4 ± 0.5	2.7 ± 0.3	3	2.6 ± 0.3	1.5 ± 0.3	1.7 ± 0.4
4	22 ± 1	9.0 ± 0.5	2.4 ± 0.2	4	7.1 ± 0.5	3.1 ± 0.2	2.3 ± 0.2
5(C)	28 ± 1	14 ± 1	2.0 ± 0.2	5	5.6 ± 0.4	7.6 ± 0.7	0.74 ± 0.08
6	39 ± 1	12 ± 1	3.4 ± 0.3	7	14.0 ± 0.7	7.4 ± 0.6	1.9 ± 0.2
7	188 ± 2	28 ± 1	6.7 ± 0.3	8	36 ± 1	23 ± 1	1.6 ± 0.1
8	249 ± 5	31 ± 1	8.0 ± 0.3				
	Kidney				Gonads		
1	10.2 ± 0.5	5.9 ± 0.9	1.7 ± 0.3	1-O	10 ± 3	5 ± 1	1.9 ± 0.5
2	15.8 ± 0.5	4.1 ± 0.4	3.9 ± 0.4	2-T	6.8 ± 0.6	4.7 ± 0.4	1.4 ± 0.2
3	5.8 ± 0.7	3.0 ± 0.5	1.9 ± 0.4	4-T	7.3 ± 1.0	2.1 ± 0.4	3.5 ± 0.8
4	20 ± 1	4.4 ± 0.6	4.6 ± 0.7	5-T	12 ± 1	3.3 ± 0.6	3.6 ± 0.7
5	49 ± 1	9 ± 1	5.8 ± 0.7	6-O	37 ± 2	9 ± 1	4.1 ± 0.7
6	51 ± 2	10 ± 1	5.2 ± 0.6				
7	166 ± 4	30 ± 2	5.5 ± 0.4		Thyroid		
8	213 ± 6	34 ± 2	6.3 ± 0.3	1	7 ± 1	6 ± 1	1.1 ± 0.3
				3	2.6 ± 0.4	1.5 ± 0.3	1.7 ± 0.5
	Small intestine				Rib		
3	1.6 ± 0.3	1.6 ± 0.4	1.0 ± 0.3	1	58 ± 5	62 ± 5	0.94 ± 0.11
4	3.6 ± 0.3	1.2 ± 0.2	3.0 ± 0.6	2	115 ± 6	129 ± 7	0.89 ± 0.07
5	4.6 ± 0.4	3.2 ± 0.4	1.4 ± 0.2	3	85 ± 10	73 ± 12	1.2 ± 0.2
6	12.1 ± 0.8	5.5 ± 0.7	2.2 ± 0.3	4	107 ± 9	133 ± 13	0.81 ± 0.10
8	53 ± 4	14.1 ± 0.7	3.8 ± 0.3	5	160 ± 7	238 ± 12	0.67 ± 0.04
				6	107 ± 9	169 ± 17	0.63 ± 0.08
				8	137 ± 7	182 ± 6	0.75 ± 0.04
	Blood						
1	1.6 ± 0.2	2.8 ± 0.4	0.6 ± 0.1				
3	0.24 ± 0.04	1.2 ± 0.2	0.20 ± 0.05				
4	0.32 ± 0.05	0.8 ± 0.1	0.40 ± 0.09				
6	1.8 ± 0.1	2.1 ± 0.3	0.9 ± 0.1				

C—Carcinoma present; O—ovary; T—testis.
Errors are one standard deviation counting error.

The order of listing is the same as that used in Table 1; lower to higher caribou consumption. The concentrations are based upon fresh weight for the soft tissue and defat weight for the rib samples. The uncertainties shown are for a one standard deviation counting error.

The values observed in the samples from the Alaskan subjects, #1 and #2, who had eaten no caribou meat are within the normal range of values reported for unexposed populations.[8,20,21] The lower lung and rib levels reported for #1 are probably due to her young age, 6 yr. Hence, if these two sets of tissues may be assumed typical, then the [210]Pb–[210]Po body burden of an Alaskan whose diet does not include caribou or reindeer meat is similar to that of individuals residing in the conterminous United States.

The ^{210}Pb and [210]Po tissue concentrations of subject #3, who ate caribou meat while in Barrow but none during the last 3 yr while living in Anchorage, are somewhat less but not significantly different from those of unexposed U.S. residents.[20,21] As HILL has reported high ^{210}Pb levels in human bone samples from northern Canada,[8] and considering the 2400-day half-life of ^{210}Pb in the skeleton,[13] it was somewhat surprising, if the dietary information is correct, that the bone level in this case is not higher than that observed. Subjects #4 and #5, who occasionally included caribou meat in their diet, contained significantly higher concentrations of [210]Po in the kidney and liver samples and possibly in the testes of the latter. The concentration of ^{210}Pb in the rib sample of #5 is high with respect to the other rib samples measured; however, it does fall within the concentration range reported by HOLTZMAN for an unexposed population.[21]

The results showed significantly higher levels of [210]Po in the soft tissues of subjects considered to be caribou or reindeer meat eaters. The concentration of [210]Po in tissues of subjects #6, #7 and #8 were about 4, 14 and 18 times, respectively, the values reported for tissues of an unexposed population.[8,20,21] Smoking data are not available for these Alaskans; however, their [210]Po lung concentrations are significantly higher than observed even in the lung of cigarette smokers.[20,22] The results in Table 2 also show, except for bone, a general increase in the [210]Po concentration with consumption of caribou or reindeer meat.

Subject #7 ate caribou regularly in winter, and, as he died on December 19, had included caribou meat in his diet for 3–4 months prior to death. Subject #6 included caribou meat in her diet a few times each month, while #8 ate reindeer regularly until 3 months prior to his death, during which time he had eaten none. It is quite interesting that although these three subjects had elevated [210]Po soft tissue levels, their ^{210}Pb bone concentrations do not show a proportional increase, and fall within the range reported by HOLTZMAN for concentrations observed in human bone samples of residents of the conterminous United States.[21] It has been reported that although caribou bones, liver and kidney contain high concentrations of ^{210}Pb,[8] the concentration in the meat is low, 5–16 pCi/kg,[6] and not much different from that observed for beef in the conterminous United States.[21] Consequently, unless the subject had consumed an extract of the caribou bone or a soft tissue which concentrates ^{210}Pb, as liver or kidney, the ^{210}Pb skeletal burden would probably not be expected to be much higher than for individuals who consumed no caribou meat.

The [210]Po/^{210}Pb activity ratio exceeds one and is generally much greater in soft tissues of the subjects who ate caribou or reindeer meat. Similar results were recently reported by KAURANEN and MIETTINEN for reindeer breeders living in Lapland.[23] These high activity ratios are especially significant in the case of the lung for which activity ratios of less than one are usually observed.[20] Since the ground-level air concentration of ^{210}Pb is about 10 times greater than [210]Po,[24] these results suggest exposure by a route other than inhalation and by a source containing [210]Po in excess of [210]Pb. These observations support the conclusion that caribou or reindeer meat is the principal source of [210]Po for this population.

When large quantities of ^{210}Pb are ingested, it is concentrated in the skeleton with an effective half-life of about 2400 days.[23] During this time, the [210]Po grows into near radioactive equilibrium with the ^{210}Pb and serves as a reservoir for other body compartments.[25] That is, some [210]Po is translocated from the skeleton to other body tissues which sustains the

[210]Po in the tissues for much longer times than is reflected by the effective half-life of the particular organ. In the case of the caribou meat eaters as observed here, only [210]Po was ingested in larger than "normal" amounts. Consequently, there is no skeletal reservoir of [210]Po supported by ^{210}Pb, and once the subject ceases to eat caribou or reindeer, the excess [210]Po is excreted quite rapidly from the soft tissues of the body. For example, the ICRP lists the effective half-lives of [210]Po in liver, kidney and spleen as 32, 46 and 42 days, respectively.[13] This probably explains why the body burden appears "normal" for subject #3 who ate caribou regularly while residing at Barrow, but not while residing in Anchorage during the three years preceding death. Except for the concentrations in the kidney and liver which appear to be significantly higher than normal, the same reasoning can explain the apparent "normal" [210]Po concentrations in tissues of subjects #4 and #5. In addition, the [210]Po tissue concentration of subject #8 who ate reindeer regularly until three months before his death was undoubtedly much higher while eating caribou than was observed at the time of his death.

The body burden of [210]Po was estimated for subject #8 by summing the products of the concentration observed in each tissue multiplied by the tissue mass, based on the 70 kg "standard man".[13] On this basis, approximately 60 % of the total body mass was analyzed. The concentration in the remaining 40 % was assumed equal to that in muscle. The [210]Po body burden of this subject, so calculated, was estimated at death to be 1.7 nCi. Taking $\frac{1}{10}$ the ICRP recommended value for an occupational exposed population as the maximum permissible body burden for the general population, the estimated body burden at death, 1.7 nCi, is about one-half the maximum burden if the spleen is assumed the critical organ.[13]

If it is assumed that the [210]Po is distributed uniformly within the organ and if 10 is used as the RBE for [210]Po alpha particles, then the dose rate in mrem/year is numerically equivalent to the concentration of [210]Po in the units of pCi/kg of tissue. Consequently, the dose rates delivered by [210]Po to these tissues may be read directly from Table 2. The soft tissues which contain the higher levels, kidney and liver, are exposed to only a few hundred mrem/year. Although these dose rates may be smaller than previously estimated for those eating caribou meat, it should be remembered that, except for #7, the subjects available for this investigation were not eating caibou or reindeer meat on a daily basis at the time of their death. Assuming the effective half-life of [210]Po in the liver and kidney as 32 days and 46 days, respectively, the concentration of [210]Po in these two tissues of subject #8 three months prior to this death when he is reported to have stopped eating caribou meat was about 1780 pCi/kg and 840 pCi/kg, respectively. This corresponds to a dose rate of about two and 1 rem/yr, respectively, if the assumptions mentioned above are correct.

In making the above extrapolation to estimate the tissue concentration 3 months prior to death, it was assumed that the metabolism during the terminal 3 months of illness was normal, the diet during this interval contained no food with abnormally high levels of [210]Po, and that the biological parameters given by ICRP for [210]Po are accurate. The first assumption may not be true and the [210]Po excretion rate may have been different than that of a healthy person. It is, however, unlikely that this individual consumed food during hospitalization which contained high concentrations of [210]Po, and the ICRP values, although possibly requiring some revision, are the best presently available. Consequently, the person who consumes caribou meat daily will probably receive larger dose rates from the [210]Po during the time of ingestion than is indicated by the results shown in Table 2. Tissue levels for such individuals would be extremely valuable; however, autopsies are rarely performed on subjects of this population, and to obtain autopsy tissue samples will be extremely difficult.

Lichens and caribou

In order to determine if thermonuclear explosions in the arctic contributed significantly to the ^{210}Pb levels in the arctic ecosystem, samples of lichen and caribou (*Rangifer tarandus*) bones which had been collected before the advent of nuclear testing in the arctic (1951), were analyzed for ^{210}Pb and [226]Ra. The collection data and analytical results for the lichen samples and caribou bones are given in Tables 3 and 4, respectively. The ^{210}Pb results have been corrected for radioactive decay to reflect the concentrations at the time of collection and the ^{210}Pb, contributed by the [226]Ra since the time of collection, has been subtracted.

The ^{210}Pb levels in 14 Alaskan lichen samples collected over the last 8 yr have been reported.[7,9,26] These varied from 3.44 to 69 pCi/g dry weight with an average of 13 ± 8 pCi/g (S.D.). The data in Table 4 indicate that lichens collected prior to 1951 had ^{210}Pb concentrations ranging from 3.41 to 34.5 pCi/g dry weight with an average of 16 ± 12 pCi/g (S.D.). Thus, there was no apparent increase in ^{210}Pb concentration due to nuclear testing activities. Further, the range of values (9.68–39.5 pCi/g) for lichen samples collected at Anaktuvuk Pass in 1949 bracket the 14.9 pCi/g recently reported from the same area.[9]

Table 3. *Concentrations of* [210]Pb *and* [226]Ra *in Alaskan lichen samples collected before* 1951

Sample	Location	Date collected	[210]Pb, *pCi/g†	[226]Ra, pCi/g†
Cetraria islandica	Point Barrow 71°19′N, 56°40′W	1948	17.3 ± 0.2	0.050 ± 0.011
Cetraria richardsonii	Point Barrow 71°19′N, 56°40′W	1948	12.2 ± 0.1	0.045 ± 0.010
Alectoria nitidula +*Cladinia* sp.	Anaktuvuk Pass 68°10′N, 51°54′W	1949	35.0 ± 0.2	0.043 ± 0.010
Sphaerophorus globosus	Anaktuvuk Pass 68°10′N, 51°54′W	1949	9.68 ± 0.12	0.125 ± 0.009
Parmelia omphalodes	Anaktuvuk Pass 68°10′N, 51°54′W	1949	39.5 ± 0.2	0.028 ± 0.004
Cetraria delisei	Wainwright 70°39′N, 160°W	1949	12.2 ± 0.1	0.034 ± 0.011
Cladonia subulata	Cape Nome 64°28′N, 165°W	1923	7.30 ± 0.10	0.122 ± 0.008
Cladonia uncialis	Noorvik-on Kobuk River 66°49′N, 161°6′W	1923	3.41 ± 0.06	0.032 ± 0.006
Cladonia cenotea	Cape Nome 64°28′N, 165°W	1923	6.2 ± 0.10	0.031 ± 0.006

* Activity corrected to date of collection and the [226]Ra contribution subtracted.
† Dry weight (dried at 90°C for 24 hr).

Table 4. *Concentrations of* [210]Pb *and* [226]Ra *in caribou bone collected before* 1951

Sample number	Location collected	Date collected	Age	Bone type	[210]Pb(pCi/g)*	[226]Ra(pCi/g)
OC-01	Longhead Island 77°20′N, 105°W	8–16	Adult	Metatarsal	15.4 ± 0.2	0.21 ± 0.01
OC-02	Ellesmere Island 78°3′N, 85°W	3–35	Adult	Occipital	8.08 ± 0.13	0.25 ± 0.01
OC-03	Teslin Dist., Yukon Terr. 60°2′N, 132°50′W	11–12	Adult	Manible	5.4 ± 0.17	0.24 ± 0.01
OC-04	Nettilling Lake, Baffinland 66°26′N, 71°W	8–25	Fawn	Ulna	1.51 ± 0.08	0.065 ± 0.006
OC-05	Near George R., Quebec 53°30′N, 66°12′W	9–49	Fawn	Scapula	2.08 ± 0.12	0.11 ± 0.01

* Activity corrected to date of collection and the [226]Ra contribution subtracted.

44

Table 5. A comparison of the ^{210}Pb content in old and recent caribou bones

Latitude	Concentration in recent (1965–1966) caribou bones (pCi ^{210}Pb/g)[6]	Concentration in pre-1951 caribou bones from Table 4 (pCi ^{210}Pb/g)
<60°N	Range: 2.1–5.6 (14)	2.1 (fawn)
	Mean: 3.1 ± 0.4	
60°–65°N	Range: 2.4–7.5 (26)	5.4
	Mean: 4.5 ± 0.4	
>65°N	Range: 4.9–13.1 (15)	15.4, 8.1
	Mean: 7.6 ± 0.6	1.5 (fawn)

Note: (a) The number of caribou are given in parentheses
(b) The uncertainties are the standard deviations of the mean.

The next step in the arctic food chain is caribou, which should also reflect higher levels of ^{210}Pb after 1951 if nuclear testing contributed substantially to the ^{210}Pb levels in the arctic environment. The ^{210}Pb results for the pre-1951 caribou bone samples given in Table 4 are compared in Table 5 to adult caribou bone samples which were collected during 1965–1966.[6] Due to a possible increase in the ^{210}Pb bone concentration with increasing latitude,[6] the results in Table 5 are arranged in three groups according to latitude. Except for sample OC-05, a fawn, the results of the pre-1951 samples are within the range of values reported for the recent samples.

As it has been reported that the ^{210}Pb skeletal burden of fawns is only about one-half that found in the skeleton of the adult,[6] the two samples from fawns, OC-04 and OC-05, are undoubtedly low relative to adult caribou from the same areas. As in the case for lichen samples, there does not appear to be any substantial increase in the ^{210}Pb skeletal burden of caribou following the advent of nuclear testing in the arctic. Consequently, it seems unlikely that arctic testing of nuclear weapons has had any significant effect on the amount of ^{210}Pb in the arctic ecosystem.

SUMMARY

Although there were relatively few tissue samples available for study, the results indicate that caribou or reindeer meat is the principal source of ^{210}Po for Alaskan residents, and that, in general, the intake of ^{210}Pb and ^{210}Po by inhalation is about the same as in the conterminous United States. In addition, it was illustrated in the case of these subjects that consumers of caribou meat may ingest large quantities of ^{210}Po unsupported by its parent, ^{210}Pb. This produces high ^{210}Po body burdens only as long as the subject continues to eat caribou or reindeer meat, and when the meat is eliminated from the diet the ^{210}Po will be excreted within a relatively short period and the body burden will approach that of an unexposed person.

The ^{210}Pb concentrations in lichen and caribou bone samples collected before 1951 were comparable to concentrations in similar samples recently collected. The data tend to discount the importance of nuclear testing in the arctic as a significant source of ^{210}Pb.

Acknowledgement—The authors thank Peter Jatlow, Alaskan Native Medical Center, Anchorage and D. J. Weider, Alaskan Native Hospital, Kotzebue, for supplying the tissue samples; Mason Hale, Smithsonian Institution, Washington, D.C., for the pre-1951 lichen samples; P. M. Youngman, National Museum of Canada, Ottawa, for the pre-1951 caribou samples; and B. Kahn, of this laboratory, for helpful suggestions during the preparation of this paper.

REFERENCES
1. A. R. Schulert, *Science* **136**, 146 (1962).
2. D. G. Watson, W. C. Hanson and J. J. Davis, *Science* **144**, 1005 (1964).
3. W. C. Hanson and H. E. Palmer, *Trans. N. Am. Wildl. Conf.* **29**, 215 (1964).
4. W. C. Hanson and H. E. Palmer, *Health Phys.* **11**, 1401 (1965).
5. W. C. Hanson, *Science* **153**, 525 (1966).
6. R. L. Blanchard and J. W. Kearney, *Environ. Sci. Technol.* **1**, 932 (1967).
7. R. B. Holtzman, *Nature Lond.*, **210**, 1094 (1966).

8. C. R. Hill, *Nature, Lond.* **208,** 423 (1965).
9. T. M. Beasley and H. E. Palmer, *Science* **152,** 1062 (1966).
10. K. Z. Morgan, W. S. Snyder and M. R. Ford, *Health Phys.* **10,** 151 (1964).
11. *Radiol. Health Rep.* **7,** 675 (1966).
12. C. R. Hill, *Science* **152,** 1261 (1966).
13. I.C.R.P. Committee II on Permissible Dose for Internal Radiation (1959), *Health Phys.* **3,** (1960).
14. Z. Jaworowski, *Nature, Lond.* **212,** 886 (1966).
15. W. L. Minto, *Biological Studies with Polonium, Radium, and Plutonium,* (Edited by R. M. Fink) p. 15. McGraw-Hill, New York (1950).
16. S. C. Black, *Health Phys.* **7,** 87 (1961).
17. A. Martin, *Health Phys.* **13,** 1348 (1967).
18. H. F. Lucas, ANL-6297, 55 (1961).
19. R. L. Blanchard, *Environmental Health Series,* U.S. Public Health Service, 999-RH-9 (1964).
20. R. L. Blanchard, *Health Phys.* **13,** 625 (1967).
21. R. B. Holtzman, *Health Phys.* **9,** 385 (1963).
22. J. B. Little, E. P. Radford, H. L. McCombs and V. R. Hunt, *N. Eng. J. Med.* **273,** 1343 (1965).
23. R. Kauranen and J. K. Miettinen, *Health Phys.* **16,** 287 (1969).
24. W. M. Burton and N. G. Stewart, *Nature, Lond.* **186,** 584 (1960).
25. R. B. Holtzman, *Health Phys.* **10,** 763 (1964).
26. R. L. Blanchard, *Radioecological Concentration Processes: Proc. Intern. Symp.* Stockholm, April 25–29, 1966 (Edited by B. Aberg and F. P. Hungate) pp. 281–296. Pergamon Press, New York (1967).

Measurement of lead-210 in surface air
and precipitation

By L. U. JOSHI, C. RANGARAJAN and Smt. SARADA GOPALAKRISHNAN, *Health Physics*

1. Introduction

In a previous publication (Rangarajan *et al.*, 1967) data on lead-210 concentrations in ground level air and precipitation at a few stations in India were presented. Therein, it was pointed out that lead-210 concentrations undergo a seasonal variation with maximum values in winter and minimum values during the summer. This was noted at Bombay and to a lesser extent at Srinagar where the variation was not so pronounced as at Bombay. It was also suggested that this seasonal variation which differed in the time of occurrence of the peak values from fission products like cesium-137 originating from the stratosphere, seemed to correlate very well with ground level radon values. In this paper extensive measurements on lead-210 made since then at the various stations listed in Table 1 are presented and their relations with other atmospheric activities like radon, fission products, etc., discussed. Activities in rainwater and their relations to air concentrations have also been explored.

2. Experimental methods

The techniques of sample collection and radioactivity measurements have already been described in detail (Rangarajan *et al.*, 1968,

Vohra *et al.*, 1966, Joshi *et al.*, 1968). The sampling volume of ground level radioactive dust collection is of the order of 50×10^3 cubic meters at Bombay and about one-tenth of this at the other stations. The Hollingsworth and Vose H-70 filters used for sampling are ashed at low temperatures (less than 400°C) prior to chemical analysis. The ashed samples along with lead carrier are digested in aqua regia and then taken in 1.5 M hydrochloric acid. These samples are then passed through anion-exchange resin Dowex-1 × 8% (50–100 mesh). The maximum adsorption of lead takes place in this acid concentration. The adsorbed lead is then eluted with 8 M hydrochloric acid. It is finally precipitated as lead sulphate and counted (Joshi *et al.*, 1967). The counting of daughter product bismuth-210 and its build-up with a half-life of 5.0 days enables the samples to be checked as well as the activity to be assayed. End-window geiger counters with a back-ground of five counts per minute are used for the beta counting of the samples. With this system, samples can be counted to an accuracy better than ±5% s.d.

Rainwater collections are made in stainless steel funnels (12" diameter) and polythene vessels. The monthly collections of rainwater are pooled together depending on the amount of rainfall to give detectable activity. Yearly

Table 1. *List of radioactivity monitoring stations in India*

Station	Altitude (Meters)	Latitude	Longitude	Type of sampling for lead-210 analysis
1. Srinagar	1598	34°06′ N	74°55′ E	Rainwater and monthly air filter analysis
2. Delhi	219	28°45′ N	77°20′ E	Do.
3. Gangtok	2000	27°12′ N	88°23′ E	Rainwater analysis. Air filter data not presented.
4. Calcutta	Sea level	22°34′ N	88°25′ E	Rainwater and monthly air filter analysis.
5. Nagpur	311	21°12′ N	79°04′ E	Do.
6. Bombay	Sea level	18°57′ N	72°55′ E	Do.
7. Bangalore	922	12°57′ N	77°30′ E	Rainwater and half-yearly air filter analysis.
8. Ootacamund	2235	11°23′ N	76°40′ E	Do.

average specific activities and depositions only are reported here. The evaporated residues of the rain samples are chemically treated as for filter ash and counted.

3. Results

Fig. 1 gives the lead-210 concentrations in air at Bombay and Srinagar from 1962 to the middle of 1966. These are a continuation of the data previously given (Rangarajan *et al.*, 1968) up-dated to the middle of 1966. Radon concentrations at Bombay not reported earlier are also included from the end of 1965 when sampling for radon was started. The radon activity is measured through its solid daughter products assuming equilibrium with radon. In view of the uncertainty in this as well as in the

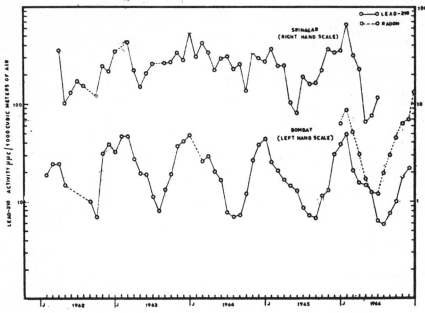

Fig. 1. Lead-210 (Ra-D) activity in ground level air at Bombay and Srinagar.

48

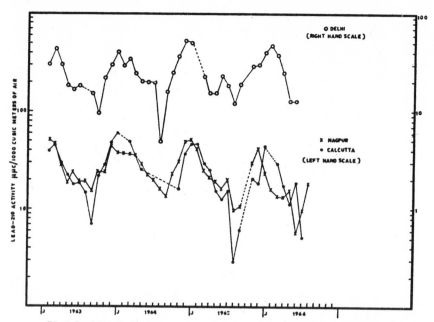

Fig. 2. Lead-210 (Ra-D) activity in ground level air at Calcutta, Nagpur and Delhi.

possibility that filter collection efficiency for the daughter products is not 100%, radon concentrations are given in relative units but if radon is in equilibrium and filter collection efficiency is taken as 100%, one unit would correspond to one micro-microcurie per cubic meter of air. The uncertainties in radon measurements are unlikely to affect the following discussions as will be shown later.

Lead-210 activities measured in surface air at three other stations, viz., Nagpur, Calcutta and Delhi are shown in Fig. 2, from 1963 onwards. These results are also based on analysis of monthly pooled filter collections as at Bombay and Srinagar.

The latitudinal variation of the average yearly concentration of lead-210 in surface air and precipitation are shown in Fig. 3 for the years 1962 to 1966. Data from two other stations, viz., Bangalore and Ootacamund are also included. The activities in the case of these two stations are based on a half-yearly sample analysis. The precipitation activities have been calculated from the total yearly deposition of lead-210 and the yearly rainfall from all the

eight stations of the sampling network (Table 1). The total yearly deposition of lead-210 is summarized in Table 2.

4. Discussion of results

Seasonal variations in surface air activity

The data on air concentration of lead-210 at the stations given in Figs. 1 and 2 show that there is a seasonal variation in activity, the maximum concentration being reached in the winter months of November, December and January and the minimum values in July and August. This seasonal cycle is observed at all the five stations although it is not as pronounced at Srinagar as at the more southerly stations. (Results for another station—Gangtok—which also shows similar seasonal variation are not reported here as the values are not yet finalised).

The climatic and other reasons for this seasonal variation can be discussed on the basis of the possible sources of lead-210 in ground level air. Ground level activity could be due to local radon diffusing from the soil or it could originate

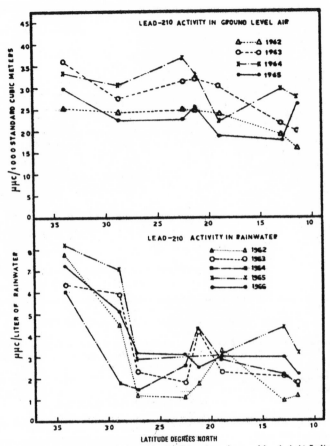

Fig. 3. Latitudinal variation of lead-210 in rain and ground level air in India.

from the upper troposphere and stratosphere where lead-210 has been sampled in significant quantities (Peirson *et al.*, 1966). The behaviour of a stratospheric source diffusing to ground level is well illustrated by the measurements on the cesium-137 activity in surface air (Rangarajan *et al.*, 1968). If lead-210 were originating from the stratosphere its peak values are likely to be observed during the spring months along with maximum values of cesium-137 in April (Rangarajan, *et al.*, 1968) rather than two to three months earlier as is the actual case. On the other hand the agreement with radon is very close as shown in Fig. 1. The possible errors

in radon measurements such as nonequilibrium with radon daughters and lesser filter collection efficiencies are unlikely to result in such close agreement between radon and lead-210. The H-70 filter used is reported (Lockhart, *et al.*, 1964) to have an efficiency of nearly 95% for radium (B + C) aerosols and disequilibrium with radon daughters is not significant as what is measured is the radon daughter concentrations which actually decay to lead-210. Hence it may be concluded that lead-210 in surface air is mainly controlled by radon concentrations, at least in continental areas.

Two reasons can be advanced for the observed

50

Station	Year				
	1962	1963	1964	1965	1966
Srinagar	4.87	4.98	2.93	5.36	6.48
	(625.2)	(782.0)	(692.0)	(653.0)	(889.9)
Delhi	2.60	4.85	2.16	2.19	3.31
	(577.2)	(817.5)	(1233.1)*	(420.5)*	(650.2)
Gangtok	3.77	8.96	3.40	4.17	10.76
	(3170.4)	(3827.4)*	(2401.2)*	(2466.0)*	(3399.3)*
Calcutta	1.32	3.03	3.85	—	3.25
	(1158.0)	(1678.0)	(1485.0)		(1025.7)*
Nagpur	2.25	3.86	2.66	—	2.17
	(1258.8)	(932.6)	(849.9)*		(858.9)
Bombay	7.50	5.12	5.24	8.66	5.79
	(2227.0)	(2229.0)	(1798.8)*	(2626.1)	(1952.0)
Bangalore	1.03	2.09	2.60	3.06	3.04
	(1052.7)	(1040.6)	(1191.6)	(692.0)	(1021.0)*
Ootacamund	1.77	2.12	3.19	2.14	3.12
	(1509.6)	(1190.0)	(1835.0)	(676.6)*	(1416.6)*

* The rainfall for these years is the total for the sampling months only but is greater than 80 % of the total annual precipitation.

annual variation in radon (and lead-210) concentrations in surface air.

A shift in surface winds from continental to maritime such as occurs when the north-east winds change into the powerful south-west monsoon over the Indian continent could result in a seasonal variation. The monsoon winds, due to lack of replenishment of radon diffusing from soil in their path across the oceans may be less radioactive than winds which have travelled over large land masses. However, the onset of the monsoon occurs some time during the period April–May when lead-210 levels have already decreased to significantly lower values compared to peak concentrations. This makes it rather difficult to correlate the fall in activity after the peak values with the onset of the south-west monsoon winds.

The occurence of frequent inversion conditions during winter could also result in high radon concentrations. Gale *et al.* (1958), found that average monthly radon concentrations showed significant correlation with the average potential temperature gradient during the period of their measurements for one year in the United Kingdom. The presence of the winter maximum at all the stations—coastal as well as inland—suggests that this could be a major factor in the seasonal variation although the effect of air mass movements cannot be ruled out. (Part of the reason for the seasonal variation not being so pronounced at Srinagar could be the lesser prevalence of the monsoon there.)

Latitudinal variation of activity

The data given in Fig. 3 shows a trend towards an increase in the specific activity of rains at high latitude stations like Srinagar although this is not so clear in the air activity data. The climate of this station (Srinagar) differs in several respects from the other lower latitude stations where precipitation is mostly in summer during monsoon when air activity—both natural and bomb produced—are at a minimum. At Srinagar, however, there is both winter and summer rains which are mostly not connected with the monsoon cycle. This difference in the precipitation system is apparently reflected in the somewhat higher specific activity at Srinagar. A similar difference in specific activity in rain was observed in the case of cesium-137 which was also attributed to the difference in the precipitation systems (Rangarajan *et al.*, 1968) between the northern stations particularly Srinagar and the other low latitude stations. In view of these results it is concluded that the specific activity of precipitation is sensitive to the origin and seasonal distribution of rainfall with respect to the peak values in airborne activity.

The general level of activities given here for India may be compared with activities in the temperate latitudes as reported by other laboratories. Airborne lead-210 activities in India vary from about 10–50 micro-microcuries per thousand cubic meters as shown in Figs. 1 to 3, while in precipitation the activities are of the order of 1–10 micro-microcuries per litre. In general the values given here are considerably higher than the activities in the U.K. (Peirson et al., 1966) of 1–10 micro-microcuries per kg of air but show agreement with the values given by Patterson (Patterson et al., 1964) for the U.S. of 3–30 micro-microcuries per thousand cubic meters and by Shleien (Shleien et al., 1967) for Massachusetts, U.S. of 4–40 micro-microcuries per thousand cubic meters. These differences can possibly be explained by the prevalence of maritime winds over islands like the U.K. and the presence of large land masses and high radioactive areas in the other case. The deciding factor seems to be the previous path of the air masses being sampled which determines their radioactive content.

5. Acknowledgements

Our thanks are due to Dr. K. G. Vohra, Head, Air Monitoring Section under whose guidance this work was carried out. We are grateful to Dr. A. K. Ganguly, Head, Health Physics Division for his encouragement. We also thank the following institutions for their help in the collection of samples: (1) Regional Meteorological Centres of the India Meteorological Department at Bangalore, Calcutta, New Delhi, Gangtok, Nagpur and Srinagar and (2) Cosmic Ray Research Laboratory of the Tata Institute of Fundamental Research at Ootacamund.

REFERENCES

Gale, H. J. & Peaple, L. H. J. 1958. Measurements on the near-ground radon concentrations on the A.E.R.E. Airfield, AERE HP/R 2381.

Joshi, L. U. & Mahadevan, T. N. 1967. Radiochemical determination of lead-210 concentrations in ground level air in India. Proceedings of the Nuclear and Radiation Chemistry Symposium, Poona.

Joshi, L. U. & Mahadevan, T. N. 1968. Seasonal variation of radium-D (Lead-210) in ground level air in India. Health Physics, 15, 67–71.

Lockhart, L. B. & Patterson, R. L. 1964. Characteristics of air filter media used for monitoring airborne radioactivity, NRL Report 6054.

Patterson, R. L. & Lockhart, L. B. 1964. Geographical distribution of lead-210 (Ra-D) in the ground-level air. The natural radiation environment. The University of Chicago press, Chicago, 383–392.

Peirson, D. H., Cambray, R. S. & Spicer, G. S. 1966. Lead-210 and polonium-210 in the atmosphere, Tellus 18, 427–433.

Rangarajan, C., Sarada, G., Sadasivan, S. & Chitale, P. V. 1968. Atmospheric and precipitation radiovity in India, Tellus 20, 269–283.

Shleien, B., Cochran, J. A., Benander, L., Bernard, L. L., Lutz., J. D. & Friend, A. G. 1967. Atmospheric radioactivity analysis and instrumentation, status report III, National Centre for Radiological Health, Public Health Service, U.S. Department of Health, Education and Welfare.

Vohra, K. G., Rangarajan, C., Sarada, G., Sadasivan, S. & Chitale, P. V. 1966. Measurements on airborne and surface fallout radioactivity in India from nuclear weapon tests, Atomic Energy Establishment Trombay (India) Report AEET-247.

ИЗМЕРЕНИЯ ИНТЕНСИВНОСТИ ВЫПАДЕНИЯ ОСАДКОВ И АКТИВНОСТИ Pb-210 В ПРИЗЕМНОМ СЛОЕ ВОЗДУХА

В данной работе проведено исследование и представлены данные об активности Pb-210 в приземном слое атмосферы и интенсивности выпадения осадков в ряде районов Индии, находящихся в пределах полосы широт от 11° до 34° с. ш. Сезонные изменения уровней активности, максимум которой приходится на зимний период, наблюдались в нескольких районах. Время распространения максимума активности Pb-210 отличается от времени распространения, соответствующего стратосферному Cs-137, но в целом согла-суется с уровнями радона. Поэтому делается заключение, что активность Pb-210, (главным образом, контролируется активностью радона в приземном слое воздуха. Обсуждаются возможные причины максимальной активности радона в зимний период. Рассматривается широтное изменение активности Pb-210 и его возможные причины. Уровни активности Pb-210 в Индии сравниваются с величинами, представленными другими лабораториями в умеренных широтах.

Investigations on ^{210}Pb Concentrations in Various Regions of India

L. U. Joshi
C. Rangarajan
Smt. Sarada Gopalakrishnan

(*Received* 23 *February* 1970; *in revised form*
16 *July* 1970)

Introduction

WE HAVE been carrying out extensive measurements of ^{210}Pb in air and precipitation at a number of stations in India as a preliminary to the assessment of its radiological significance in the Indian environment. In previous publications[1-3] data on the seasonal and geographical variations of ^{210}Pb concentrations at some stations in India and the meteorological causes for these were discussed. Since these studies had indicated the possibility that ^{210}Pb levels could be mainly controlled by the prevailing radon concentrations, measurements of ^{210}Pb were continued at the other stations, viz. Gangtok, Nainital and Thumba to explore · the possibility of increased ^{210}Pb levels resulting from high uranium or ^{226}Ra activity of the soil in certain parts of the country. These new measurements in relation to our previous data will be discussed.

Experimental Methods

Methods of sample collection, processing, chemical separation and counting have already been described in great detail[1,2] and will not be elaborated here. Rainwater collection is done in stainless steel vessels of 30 cm dia. and atmospheric particulates are sampled by passing air through Hollingsworth and Vose, H-70 filters using powerful blowers. The residue of rainwater after evaporation and of air filters after ashing below 400°C are subjected to radiochemical separation by Ion Exchange methods and are finally beta counted for ^{210}Bi in-growth of the lead sample. The statistical accuracy of the countings is usually better than $\pm 5\%$ standard deviation.

53

Results and Discussion

Figures 1 and 2 show the seasonal variations of ^{210}Pb at the various stations in India. Figure 3 compares the radon daughter activity with ^{210}Pb activity at Bombay. Figure 4 gives the latitudinal variation of ^{210}Pb in surface air and rainfall.

The previous findings on the spatial and seasonal variation of ^{210}Pb can be summarised as follows.

(a) ^{210}Pb in surface air undergoes a seasonal variation with max values in winter (December–February) and min values in summer (July–August). This was noted at all the stations (although not very pronounced at Srinagar) and seems to be a characteristic feature of the continent. A comparison with stratospheric ^{137}Cs showed that at the time of its spring max in April, ^{210}Pb levels had reduced significantly from the peak values 2–3 months earlier in mid-winter. This rules out the possibility of the presence of significant amounts of ^{210}Pb from upper atmosphere in the ground level air. However, radon daughter measurements made at 9.00 hr in the morning and 15.00 hr in the afternoon showed that there was a seasonal variation of radon daughters similar to ^{210}Pb with peak values in mid-winter (Fig. 3). In view of this correspondence it was postulated that ^{210}Pb levels were mainly dependent on the prevailing radon concentrations.

Meteorological data showed that the most likely reason for the seasonal variation of radon is the greater prevalence of inversion conditions in winter although a secondary cause could be the change of surface winds from the continental North-East monsoon to the South-West monsoon in summer.

(b) Studies on the latitudinal variations of specific activity showed that air concentrations (Fig. 4) at the stations previously measured were not significantly different, varying by about 50% from an average of about 25 pCi/1000 standard m^3. A more significant variation of the specific activity of rainfall was however noted (Fig. 4) with a sharp increase towards higher latitudes. This was attributed mainly to the difference in the precipitation system at high latitudes where the winter rains due to the 'Mediterranean Disturbances' are more prominent than the summer monsoon rains. (Most of the stations at lower latitudes have no precipitation during winter when the airborne levels of radon are max.).

Recent measurements made at Gangtok, Nainital and Thumba showed, that in general, the seasonal behaviour of ^{210}Pb at Gangtok and Thumba were consistent with the basic features described above but data for Nainital did not show a pronounced variation. Limited data makes it difficult to draw any conclusion but this station is at a high altitude

54

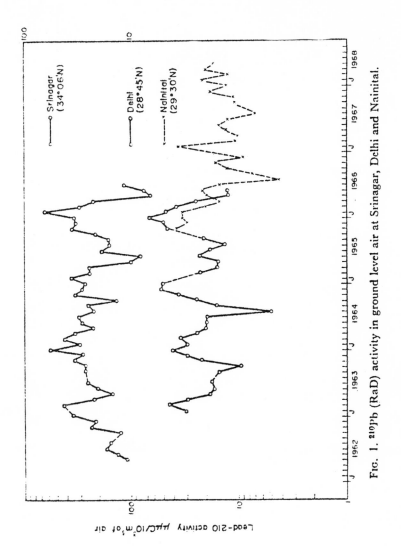

Fig. 1. ^{210}Pb (RaD) activity in ground level air at Srinagar, Delhi and Nainital.

55

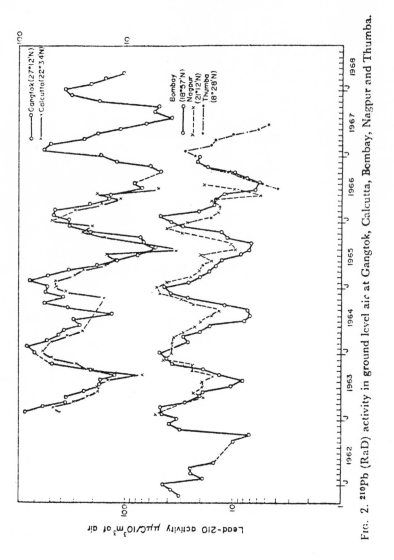

Fig. 2. ^{210}Pb (RaD) activity in ground level air at Gangtok, Calcutta, Bombay, Nagpur and Thumba.

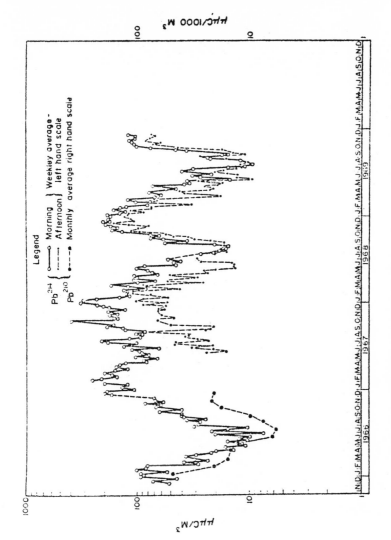

Fig. 3. ^{214}Pb (RaB) and ^{210}Pb (RaD) activity in surface air at Bombay.

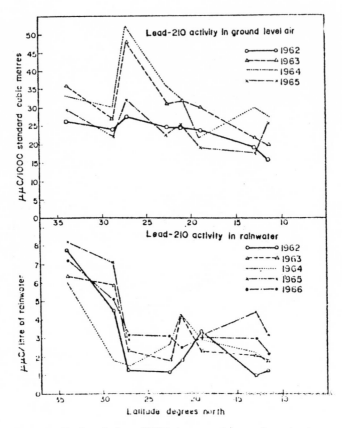

Fig. 4. Latitudinal variation of ^{210}Pb in ground level air and rain in India.

and the seasonal cycle for radon may not be very effective.

The results of Fig. 4 also show that the Gangtok values, particularly during 1963 and 1964 are higher by a factor of two compared to the other stations. From Fig. 1 it is also evident that the increase is found to be mainly during the winter months, the values during the summer months being comparable to that at the other stations.

Investigations of the likely reason for this increase led us to the conclusion that most probably the high values in winter result from meteorological conditions. Soil measurements made by MISHRA[4] showed that although ^{226}Ra at Gangtok was higher than at the other stations, the increase is not significant to explain the high ^{210}Pb levels observed. This, as well as the fact that high levels are in winter only, seems to suggest that the reason for the increased levels could be the comparatively higher stability of the lower atmosphere at Gangtok.

The possibility of enhanced body burden in view of these higher levels needs to be investigated by analysis of autopsy samples collected at Gangtok.

Acknowledgements—Our thanks are due to Dr. A. K. GANGULY, Head, Health Physics Division and to Dr. K. G. VOHRA. Head, Air Monitoring Section for their guidance and keen interest in the work.

Air Monitoring Section
Health Physics Division
Bhabha Atomic Research Centre
Trombay, Bombay-85, India

References

1. L. U. JOSHI and T. N. MAHADEVAN, *Health Phys.* **15**, 67 (1968).
2. C. RANGARAJAN, S. GOPALAKRISHNAN, S. SADASIVAN and P. V. CHITALE, *Tellus*, **XX**, 2 (1968).
3. L. U. JOSHI, C. RANGARAJAN and S. GOPALAKRISHNAN, *Tellus*, **XXI**, 1 (1969).
4. U. C. MISHRA, Unpublished data.

59

SEASONAL VARIATIONS OF RADIUM-D (LEAD-210) IN GROUND LEVEL AIR IN INDIA

L. U. JOSHI and T. N. MAHADEVAN

INTRODUCTION

LEAD-210 is formed in the atmosphere from the decay of radon gas which diffuses out from the radium in the soil. The formation of ^{210}Pb from radon gas is as given below.

$$^{226}\text{Ra} \xrightarrow[1580\,y]{\alpha} {}^{222}\text{Rn} \xrightarrow[3.8\,d]{\alpha} \text{RaA} \xrightarrow[3.05\,m]{\alpha} \text{RaB} \xrightarrow[26.8\,m]{\beta} \text{RaC}$$

$$\text{RaC} \underset{\beta}{\overset{\alpha}{\diamondsuit}} \begin{matrix} \text{RaC}'' \\ \text{RaC}' \end{matrix} \underset{\alpha}{\overset{\beta}{\diamondsuit}} \text{RaD}(^{210}\text{Pb})$$

$$^{210}\text{Pb} \xrightarrow[21\,y]{\beta} {}^{210}\text{Bi} \xrightarrow[5\,d]{\beta} {}^{210}\text{Po} \xrightarrow[140\,d]{\alpha} {}^{206}\text{Pb}\ (\text{Stable})$$

All the daughter products of radon are short-lived except ^{210}Pb and ^{210}Po.

Radon daughter products formed in the decay of radon gas condense on the aerosols present in the atmosphere and hence RaD is present in the atmospheric particulates.

Radon gas also diffuses into the upper troposphere and lower stratosphere in small quantities and has been measured there by balloons and aircrafts.[1] The daughter products of radon like RaA, RaB, etc., decay to long-lived RaD which can accumulate to some extent in the upper atmosphere from where it can be transferred to the lower atmosphere. A study of ^{210}Pb variation through the year along with fission products like ^{137}Cs which have a stratospheric origin could help in determining the origin of ^{210}Pb in the lower atmosphere and its variation with the seasons.

SAMPLE COLLECTION

The collection of air filtering samples was carried out by sucking air through Hollingsworth and Vose H-70 filter papers using powerful blowers. The volume of air sampled was about 40,000 m³ of air per month at Bombay. The daily collection was done for about 22 hr. The filter paper samples were collected every day, and the samples were pooled for 1 month. The monthly samples were ashed in a platinum crucible at 250°C.

EXPERIMENTAL

(a) The adsorption of lead on Dowex-1 × 8%, 50–100 mesh was found to be maximum near 1.5 M HCl and minimum at low hydrochloric acid concentrations and above 8 M HCl. The ashed sample with lead carrier (30 mg of lead as lead nitrate) was digested in aqua regia. The residue was dissolved in 1.5 M HCl and passed through Dowex-1. For the minimum contamination of lead the adsorbed lead was eluted with 8 M HCl and then precipitated as lead sulphate.

The lead sulphate precipitate was dissolved in ammonium acetate, and then lead was precipitated as sulphide. It was then dissolved in nitric acid and finally lead was precipitated as sulphate in which form it was counted.

(b) Some air-filter samples from Tarapur near Bombay and soil sample from Goregaon (Bombay) were used for the separation of lead

Table 3. Lead-210 activity of ground level air at Srinagar ($\mu\mu$Ci/1000 m^3)

Months	1962	1963	1964	1965	1966
January	—	—	30.4	36.6	64.6
February	—	43.4	42.3	24.7	31.0
March	35.2	22.1	33.8	24.9	22.8
April	10.1	15.0	22.5	10.2	
May	13.1	20.6	29.4	8.1	
June	17.1	25.9	30.9	18.9	
July	15.5	—	22.6	16.0	
August	—	26.7	25.8	16.5	
September	12.1	26.8	13.6	22.0	
October	24.8	34.0	33.7	36.3	
November	21.6	28.1	29.3	33.6	
December	34.7	55.0	27.1	34.9	
Average	20.5	29.8	28.5	23.6	39.4

62

Table 2. Lead-210 activity of ground level air at Bombay ($\mu\mu$Ci/1000 m^3)

Months	1961	1962	1963	1964	1965	1966
January	—	18.8	46.6	—	25.9	49.0
February	—	24.3	46.7	26.2	20.9	20.8
March	—	24.3	27.2	29.1	16.8	15.3
April	—	14.7	19.6	20.2	14.7	
May	—	—	19.0	16.7	13.0	
June	—	—	10.2	7.8	8.6	
July	—	—	8.1	7.0	7.3	
August	—	10.0	13.2	7.3	6.8	
September	—	6.9	19.0	12.0	11.4	
October	31.1	30.7	37.4	26.7	12.9	
November	38.1	38.8	41.7	38.7	30.2	
December	44.8	32.5	48.5	44.3	38.1	
Average	38.0	22.3	28.1	21.5	17.2	28.3

Table 1. *Activities of radium-D (Lead-210) and uranium from soil and air-filter samples*

Sample No.	Type of the sample	Place of collection	Period of collection	Uranium activity (dis/min)	Ra-D activity (dis/min)	Weight of the sample (g)
1(a)	Air Filter	Tarapur (S*)	March 1966	0.15	99.0	0.108
1(b)	Air Filter	Tarapur (R*)	March 1966	0.46	13.1	0.108
2(a)	Air Filter	Tarapur (S*)	April 1966	0.09	83.0	0.142
2(b)	Air Filter	Tarapur (R*)	April 1966	0.10	20.6	0.142
3(a)	Soil	Goregaon, Bombay (S*)	May 1966	0.23	2.7	1.427
3(b)	Soil	Goregaon, Bombay (R*)	May 1966	0.89	Nil	1.427

* The letters (S) and (R) in column 3 represent the soluble fraction and residue in the ammonium acetate leaching. The two parts of the each sample were used for the estimation of uranium and radium-D, respectively.

by ammonium acetate leaching. This method has removed more than 80 % of lead which was deposited on the surface of the dust particles. The remaining lead was in insoluble form and was obtained in solution by acid leaching. The soluble fraction in ammonium acetate was used for the separation of ^{210}Pb as given in (a). The insoluble fraction of the sample was digested in aqua regia and then taken in 1.5 M HCl and passed through Dowex-1. Lead was then purified as given in (a).

The effluent obtained after passing the sample in 1.5 M HCl through Dowex-1, was evaporated to dryness and taken in 8 M HCl. The solution was passed through Dowex-1. Uranium was adsorbed on the column. It was then eluted with 1.0 M HCl. The amount of uranium present in the sample was determined by fluorimetry.

The results of uranium and ^{210}Pb in soil and air-filter samples are given in Table 1.

From these results, it can be concluded that the amount of ^{210}Pb collected on air-filter from the dust particles from the soil is negligible. The ^{210}Pb collection on air-filters is therefore primarily due to the radon escape from the soil and rocks.

COUNTING

The planchet containing the sample was counted in an end-window G.M. counter (background 10.5 counts/min). The estimation of ^{210}Pb was done through the measurement of the 1.17 MeV betas of daughter product ^{210}Bi (RaE). The build up of the daughter product activity with a half-life of 5 days was followed for a period of 1 month (Fig. 1). This also gives a measure of the purity of the radio-chemical separation. The counting statistics

65

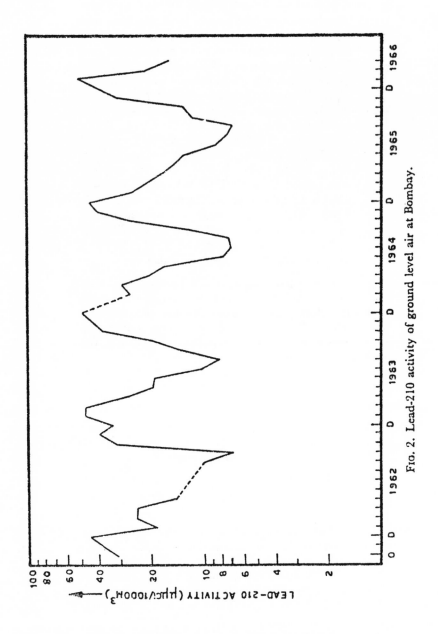

FIG. 2. Lead-210 activity of ground level air at Bombay.

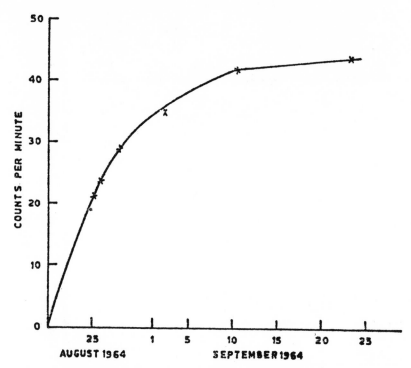

FIG. 1. Growth of RaE activity in RaD sample (Bombay airborne dust).

was better than $\pm 5\%$ standard deviation (S.D.) for all samples except a few low activity samples from Srinagar, where the sampling volume was lesser. The counting error was $\pm 7\%$ standard deviation for the samples from Srinagar.

RESULTS AND DISCUSSION

Tables 2 and 3 give the [210]Pb (RaD) activities of ground level air at Bombay and Srinagar for the periods of measurements. The levels vary from 6 $\mu\mu$Ci/1000 m³ to 60 $\mu\mu$Ci/1000 m³. The yearly averages at the two stations are also given for comparison.

The concentration of ^{210}Pb at Bombay (Fig. 2) shows a seasonal variation with maxi-

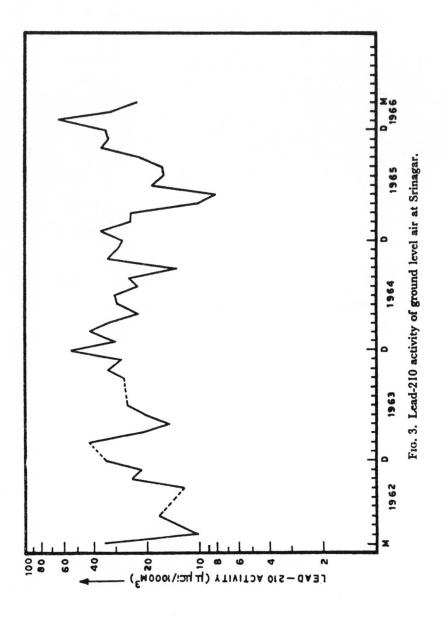

Fig. 3. Lead-210 activity of ground level air at Srinagar.

mum concentrations in winter (December–January) and minimum values in summer (July–August). The likely causes for these variations can be investigated by comparison with the concentrations of ^{137}Cs. A seasonal variation of ^{137}Cs in ground level air in India has been observed for the past several years[2] with maximum concentrations in the spring of each year and the minimum values in summer and autumn. This has been explained as being due to the enhanced transfer of stratospheric debris into the troposphere during winter and spring of each year.

Lead-210 at ground level may be due to local radon daughter product concentrations or due to ^{210}Pb which can diffuse to lower levels from the upper troposphere and stratosphere. BURTON et al.[3] has shown high concentrations of ^{210}Pb throughout the troposphere and in lower stratosphere.

However, the variation of ^{210}Pb at ground level is unlikely to be related to the seasonal variation of ^{137}Cs and other stratospheric sources for the following reasons. The maximum values of ^{210}Pb in ground level occurs 2–4 months earlier than ^{137}Cs, being mostly in December or January. The peak values in ^{137}Cs are observed during the months of March–May of each year. Secondly, the variation seems to be generally similar to radon daughter product concentration as a few preliminary measurements made in the laboratory have shown. In view of this, it is likely that the variation in ^{210}Pb concentration is purely local phenomenon related to radon daughter product build up during winter.

The Srinagar results (Fig. 3) also show a seasonal increase similar to Bombay but the variations are not as pronounced. This is likely to be due to differences in the local meteorological conditions prevalent at Srinagar compared to Bombay.

Acknowledgements—Our thanks are due to Dr. A. K. GANGULY, Head, Health Physics Division and to Dr. K. G. VOHRA, Head, Air Monitoring Section for their guidance and encouragement. We are also grateful to SHRI C. RANGARAJAN and SMT. SARADA GOPALAKRISHNAN for their help in various stages of the work.

REFERENCES

1. LESTER MACHTA and HENRY F. LUCAS, JR., *Science* 135, No. 3500, 296 (1962).
2. C. RANGARAJAN, SARADA GOPALAKRISHNAN, S. SADASIVAN and P. V. CHITALE, Measurements of airborne radioactive fallout in India, *A.E.E.T.*-208 (1965).
3. W. M. BURTON and N. G. STEWART, Radiochemical analysis of long-lived radon decay products and their use as natural atmospheric tracers, *AERE-HP/R*-2084 (1960).

Lead In The Environment

Clair C. Patterson, Ph.D.

Major changes in the course of hominid genetic
evolution during the past several million years have
been associated with important environmental
crises. In the past, the causative factor seems to
have been glacial cycles. For example, climatic
changes, the rise of seas, and shifts in populations
of flora and fauna which accompanied the retreat
of the great Illinoisian glaciers about 200,000 years
ago (figure 1) probably had something to do with
initiating the appearance and widespread dispersal
of *Homo sapiens neanderthalensis* over North
Africa, Southwest Asia, and Europe. A similar
advance of the worldwide Wisconsin glaciers (figure
1) likewise probably influenced the disappearance
of *sapiens neanderthalensis* and the appearance of
Homo sapiens sapiens. In the last two decades a
large amount of evidence and interpretation has
accumulated which clearly shows that the environmental crises caused by the retreat of the worldwide Wisconsin glaciers (figure 1) brought about
the appearance of sedentary agriculturists and hus-
bandrymen who developed, during the past 12,000
years, our civilizations.

Today a new factor operating to the same ends by changing the environment, but proceeding by different means, seems to have been forged out of the biosphere's endless searching along new paths of technological evolution, and that is engineering technology. The effect of engineering technology on the evolution of hominids cannot be predicted in detail now, but it seems evident that it will bring about the demise of *sapiens sapiens*, probably through manipulation of germ plasm and the manufacture of living brain tissue by hominines to create socio-organic entities consisting of clusters of modified hominines centering their actions about massive brains. Such "organs" and "tissues" of these entities would be dependently linked by nutrient-sensation-reward-relations.

Lead is useful for tracing this anatomy of our demise because it can be readily studied, because it was used by men throughout the last half of the post-Wisconsin urban civilization era, when the quiet gestation of engineering technology was difficult to perceive, and because its use was simply and directly related to a number of factors and activities that were important to the genesis of engineering technology.

Lead was first used about 2500 BC, at the beginning of the cupellation stage of metallurgy in Southwest Asia. By that time men were mining and smelting metal ores and they were well acquainted with the remarkable utility of bronze and the value of gold. In their attempts to smelt useful bronzes from different, abundant ores, they had finally discovered that small amounts of silver could be parted (cupelled) from lead metal which had been first smelted from lead ores. Previously, native silver had been much rarer than gold, and perhaps more esteemed. Traces of silver occur commonly in galena, an abundant lead sulfide ore, and silver production from lead ores boomed after 2500 BC. About four hundred tons of lead in oxide form were produced for every ton of silver obtained by cupellation. Lead oxide was easily converted to metal again by reduction with charcoal. With the advent of coinage in 650 BC, silver became a keystone in the founding and operation of successive civilizations and lead production rose sharply.

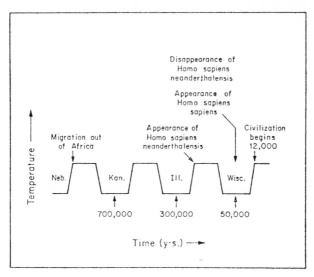

Figure 1

Worldwide glacial pulses. Such unstable climatic fluctuations have been rare in the past 1,000,000,000 years. It was uniformly warm and mild during most of that period.

During the two millenia beginning with the cupellation of silver from lead ores and ending with the commencement of coinage, men found a multitude of uses for the huge piles of lead that began to accumulate. By Classic Greek times water was being collected from lead-covered roofs, and transported through lead metal gutters to lead-lined cisterns. Stone building blocks were being held together with iron clamps embedded in lead metal that had been poured into holes drilled in the stone. Ships were being sheathed with lead metal to repel wood-worms. Salves, ointments, cosmetics, and paints were being made of lead compounds. Grape sugars boiled down in lead pots, were being added to wines to keep them from souring[1]. Lead-tin alloys were being widely used to line the inside of bronze utensils to keep copper out of foods and liquids.

Silver recovered from lead ores had a short life due to irrecoverable loss when circulating, and this factor may have been instrumental in bringing about the decline of the Roman Empire and initiating the Dark Ages in Europe. On the basis of geological and archaeological evidence and of mine production since 1800 AD for regions within the former Roman Republic and Empire, it is estimated that world silver production (essentially Roman) reached a maximum rate of about 170 tons per year at about 50 AD. Estimates can be made of the degrees of exhaustion of the lead-silver mines achieved by the Romans by comparing the depths of Roman working below the water tables in the ore deposits with the total extent of ore lodes revealed by recent mining operations. It appears that the Romans exhausted, for most practical purposes within their engineering and business capabilities, *all* the lead-silver deposits lying within the boundaries of their Empire. From a physical point of view (dated artifacts, uncertainty in degree of exhaustion, and uncertainty in production levels), the data when this occurred is uncertain within a century or so, but judging from historical evidence, it probably came at about 200 AD. Lead ore exhaustion probably was the major cause of declining silver production after that date, although the occurrence, virtually without respite during the 3rd century AD, of general anarchy and invasions within the Empire did have an adverse effect.

It is likely that the following chain of events helped in the disintegration of the Empire: the building of an economy based on the mobile exchange of silver money; lead-silver ore exhaustion; reduced silver production; reduced silver stocks because of irrecoverable loss; and economic chaos following upon the significant disappearance of silver. The rise and fall of Classic Greek civilization from 650 BC to 350 BC is linked in a similar manner to the Laurion lead mines of Attica.

Lead's link to the cores of post-Wisconsin urban civilizations by means of silver is not the only aspect of its relationship to the gestation of engineer-

74

ing technology. Lead is the most ancient, important environmental poison created by man. Many hundreds of millions of people have been affected by its toxicity during the last 4500 years, either as mining slaves, as consumers of adulterated wine and food, or as mere breathers of urban air. The magnitude of lead's toxic effect upon humanity is related to gross production. The industrial use of lead in the world reached a monumental plateau during the 1st and 2nd centuries of the Christian era. In Italy, the annual industrial use at the time amounted to nearly 0.004 ton of lead/person/year, which approximated the 0.01 ton of lead/person/year industrially used in the United States two thousand years later. World lead production declined precipitously with the fall of Rome, and then remained at a low ebb during the following six centuries. Production again began to climb slowly in Europe after the 9th century AD, when most lead mining activities shifted from holdings in the declining Byzantine Empire to virgin deposits operated by free entrepreneurs in central Europe. During the late Renaissance, world lead production finally reached the former mighty levels achieved by the Romans, after entire Indian nations became enslaved in the lead mines of Peru and Mexico. Beginning with the Industrial Revolution, world lead production climbed exponentially from 100,000 tons/yr in 1750 to 3,500,000 tons/yr in 1966. Curves illustrating the rise of world lead production with time since the Industrial Revolution are shown in figure 2.

Industrial lead enters the oceans via rivers and by atmospheric washout. Contributions from both routes have changed with time: gradually increasing during past centuries, with pollution from the atmosphere increasing abruptly during the last two decades as a consequence of a sudden growth in the rate of burning of leaded automotive fuels. The industrial use of lead is so massive today that the amount of lead mined and introduced into our relatively small urban environment each year is more than 100 times greater than the amount of natural lead leached each year from soil by streams and added to the oceans over the entire earth.

Measurements of lead in oceanic sediments and their rates of accumulation show that 1.3×10^{10}gm of dissolved lead entered the oceans per year several million years ago, while measurements of lead in rivers show that some 2.4×10^{11}gm of dissolved lead now enters the oceans. This industrial lead, plus that washed out of the air, causes high concen-

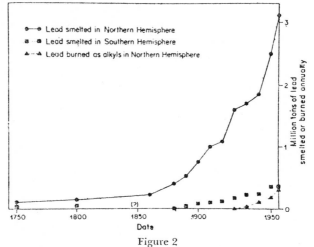

Figure 2

World lead smelter and lead alkyl production since 1750 AD. Data from Murozumi et al[2].

trations to occur in the upper, young layers of the oceans, which exceed those in the deep, ancient waters (figure 3).

This relationship is contrary to observations for other trace metals related to lead, such as barium (figure 4), where the natural distribution is controlled by organisms ingesting the metals in the upper layers, falling directly to the ocean floor, and

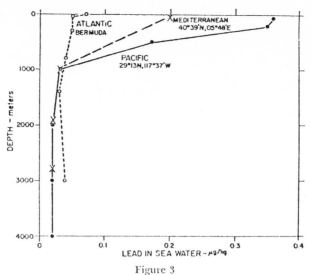

Figure 3

Lead concentration profiles in the oceans. From Chow and Patterson[3].

thus depleting the upper layers. In recent decades the massive introduction of industrial lead has swamped out this natural distribution.

The atmospheric entry of industrial lead to the seas is important today because very large amounts of lead are now burned in gasoline. This practice first began in 1924, and if it serves as an important means of introducing lead into the oceans, lead concentrations should have increased markedly in the atmosphere of the northern hemisphere after 1924. This was shown to occur by measuring increases in concentrations of lead in annual layers of snow in northern Greenland (figure 5). Concentrations of sea salts and silicate dusts did not

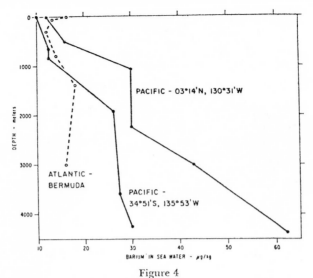

Figure 4

Barium concentration profiles in the oceans. From Chow and Patterson[3].

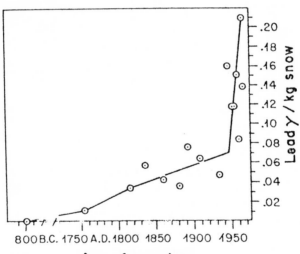

Figure 5

Lead concentration profile in snow strata of northern Greenland. From Murozumi et al[2].

78

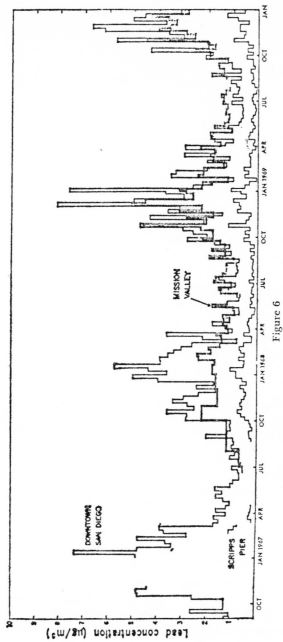

Figure 6

Concentrations of lead in the air near San Diego, California. From Chow and Earl[4].

79

change appreciably with time in the snow layers, and natural lead contributed by these materials amounted to about 0.0004 γ Pb/kg snow. At 800 BC, the analytical lead blank of 0.003 γ Pb/kg snow exceeded natural lead levels in the snow. At the beginning of the Industrial Revolution in 1750 AD, however, industrial lead concentrations had risen to about 25 times above natural levels, and this effect could be observed. By 1940 industrial lead concentrations had climbed to 175 times above natural levels. After 1940 industrial lead rose abruptly over a short interval to 500 times above natural levels. Material balance considerations indicate that this lead, deposited in Arctic regions, comprises about 1% of the leaded exhaust emissions from automobiles at temperate latitudes.

The concentration of lead in the atmosphere varies according to how close one comes to the sources, which are the cities. The approximate concentrations (in micrograms per cubic meter) are, successively: north polar regions <.0005; central ocean regions .001; U.S. countrysides .05; and U.S. cities 2.

Ventilation within cities is determined by horizontal air currents beneath inversion layer ceilings. These ceilings are elevated in the summer and are lowered in the winter, so urban atmospheric lead concentrations are higher in the winter because the volume of the city air chamber is smaller. This effect is shown in figure 6, where the cyclic rise and fall of lead over four winters in San Diego air is shown. Concentrations vary by about a factor of 4.

Most of the lead emitted as automobile exhaust consists of small, long-lived aerosols, but a portion is made up of very large particles that fall out almost immediately along roadsides. Figure 7 shows that lead concentrations in soil decrease by more than a factor of ten within about 400 meters of the road. Similar decreases in the lead contents of grasses and foliage are also observed. Ventilation reduces atmospheric lead concentrations to ambient levels within about the same distance. These characteristics are important in considering the effects upon children in schools located near freeways and upon food crops grown near highways.

It can be shown by material balance considerations that about 99% of the lead in urban atmospheres originates from automobile fuel, but isotopic tracer techniques illustrate the matter more simply and directly. Figure 8 shows the close correlation between the isotopic compositions of leads used in

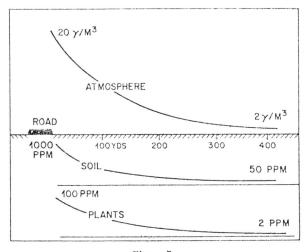

Figure 7
Lead concentrations in air, soil, and plants adjacent to a highway. Data summarized from Chow[5] and Motto et al.[6].

gasoline in various cities of the world and of leads found in the atmospheres or soils of those cities. Leads from different mines have different isotopic compositions, and these different leads are used at various locations.

Principal aspects of the pathways of lead through the human body are shown in figure 9. Typically, more than a third of the lead entering the main bloodstream originates from leaded gasolines. Much of this lead is excreted in the urine, but a part is stored in bone, where it comprises about 90% of the body burden. About 1% of the lead in the bone bank is in contact with the main bloodstream at all times and can be withdrawn to affect soft tissue.

It is observed that barium, a toxic, trace heavy metal in the calcium family of metals is rejected by plants and animals along successive steps in the food chain so that calcium in higher animals contains only one three-hundredth of the barium originally existing in soil calcium (table 1). The chemical properties of lead are so similar to barium

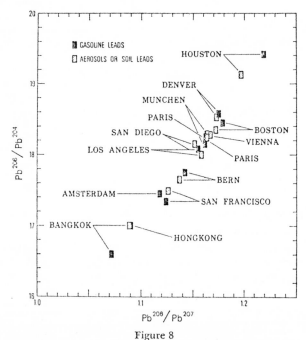

Figure 8
Correlations between the isotopic compositions of leads in gasolines with leads in local air and soil. From Chow[7].

82

in many ways that it may also be considered for some purposes a toxic, trace heavy metal member of the calcium family of metals. It is observed that calcium in the bodies of typical lead polluted Americans contains about the same proportion of lead as does calcium in soil. On the other hand, in conformity with the barium picture, it is observed that other toxic, trace heavy metals which are not used in such large quantities as lead is in the U.S.A., such as mercury and thallium, are one-hundred times less abundant in body calcium of Americans than in soil calcium. This hundred-fold discordant increase of the body burden of lead in contaminated Americans above inferred natural levels in humans is much larger than probable errors in our theoretical views on the geochemical

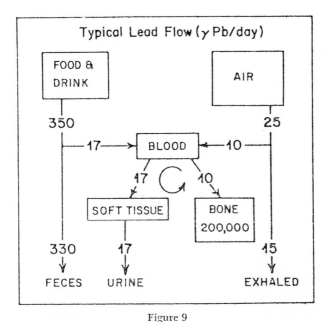

Figure 9
Principal pathways of ingested lead in the body with material balance data.

TABLE 1

ALKALINE EARTH METALS AND LEAD IN MAN AND HIS ENVIRONMENTS
(PARTS OF METAL PER MILLION PARTS OF CALCIUM).*

Metal	Atomic Weight	Earth's Crust	Terrestrial Plants	Man's Diet	Mg Metal/70 Kg Man
Ca	40	1,000,000	1,000,000	1,000,000	1,000,000
Sr	88	7,400	3,000	1,500	300
Ba	137	7,400	1,100	430	22
Pb	207	550	80	30	200**
(Estimated natural Pb levels)					2

*—From Patterson[8].   **—Observed typical value.

84

distribution of metals in the biosphere. The absolute quantities of industrial lead contamination required to produce this effect are very small and material balance calculations show that it can readily be accounted for as tiny fractions lost from various large sources of industrial lead in our urban environments.

These observations suggest that the body burdens of lead in typical urban dwellers today are several orders of magnitude above natural levels. The exposure of humans to such severe chronic lead insult probably has deleterious effects. Figure 10 shows that δ-aminolevulinic acid dehydrase, which catalyzes the formation of porphobilinogen from δ-aminolevulinic acid, is inhibited at all ranges of lead exposure in the red blood cell. It is doubtful that there is a threshold for damage, and it is believed instead that damage to humans, especially to the central nervous system, is more or less proportional to the degree of exposure.

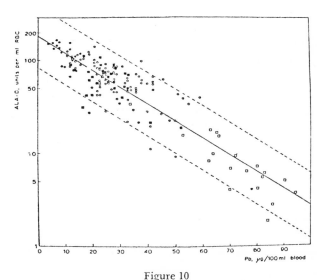

Figure 10
Relationship between blood lead levels (exposure to lead contamination) and reduction of δ-ALA dehydrase activity. After Hernberg et al[9].

Unfortunately, learning of these matters does not automatically lead to their cure because of the conflict of public and private interests that are involved. The pollution of man's environment on a worldwide scale by industrial lead has been proceeding virtually unnoticed and unchallenged for thousands of years and with an intensity which has been increasing exponentially during the last two centuries. The major factor which allowed this to happen was the simultaneous development in medicine, during the nineteenth century, of the useful and humane concept of occupational health hazard together with knowledge of the toxicity of lead. This prevented the recognition of lead as one of the first great environmental poisons because lead poisioning was relegated to the category of an occupational health hazard which seemed amenable to cure by proper care during the industrial production and manufacture of leaded materials. The seriousness of the problem of environmental pollution by industrial lead was made known recently and since that time the subject has received wide recognition, but not much has actually been accomplished, because of the massive opposition by lead producing and consuming industries to any attempts to curb the industrial production and use of lead.

References

1. Gilfillan, S. C. Lead poisoning and the fall of Rome. *Journal of Occupational Medicine* 7, 53-55, 1965.
2. Murozumi, M., T. J. Chow and C. Patterson Chemical Concentrations of Pollutant Lead Aerosols, Terrestrial Dusts and Sea Salts in Greenland and Antarctic Snow Strata. *Geochimica et Cosmochimica Acta 33* 1247-1294, 1969.
3. Chow, T. J. and C. Patterson Concentration profiles of Barium and Lead in Atlantic waters off Bermuda. *Earth and Planetary Science Letters 1*, 397-399, 1966.
4. Chow, T. J. and J. L. Earl Lead Aerosols in the Atmosphere: Increasing Concentrations. *Science 169*, 577-580, 1970.
5. Chow, T. J. Lead Accumulation in Roadside Soil and Grass. *Nature 225*, 295-296, 1970.
6. Motto, H. L., R. H. Daines, D. M. Chilko and C. K. Motto Lead in Soils and Plants: its relationship to traffic volume and proximity to highways. *Environmental Science and Technology 4*, 231-238, 1970.
7. Chow, T. J. Isotopic Identification of Industrial Pollution

Lead. 2nd International Clean Air Congress, Washington, D.C., Dec. 1970. Academic Press, New York, 1971.

8. Patterson, C. Contaminated and natural lead environments of man. *Archives of Environmental Health 11*, 344-364, 1965.

9. Hernberg, S., J. Nikkanen, G. Mellin, and H. Lilius δ-Aminolevulinic Acid Dehydrase as a Measure of Lead Exposure. *Archives of Environmental Health 21*, 140-145, 1970.

Lead and The Legislature—1971

Robert G. Oliver, B.A., LL.B.

The primary goal for State Legislators in 1971 will not be to enact entirely new laws, but rather to expedite and facilitate enforcement of existing legislation: not to fill a law-making gap, but to bridge an enforcement gap, to impart a sense of urgency to all those engaged in housing, health and child care work on both the City and State levels.

Today, there is in existence in Connecticut a basic State legislative structure, which, though imperfect, nevertheless, provides the basis for an attack upon many of the causes of lead poisoning. For example, the 1967 General Assembly adopted Public Act 743, which forbids the use of paint containing dangerous amounts of lead and other poisonous metals in interior and accessible exterior surfaces of structures housing three or more families. The same act barred use by any municipality or local housing authority of poisonous paint in any public housing projects and required the State Director of Purchase to promulgate standards for purchase of paint by the State.

Subsequently, in 1969, Public Act 533 required all paint cans sold in Connecticut after January 1, 1970, to contain the following warning label:

'CAUTION—CONTAINS LEAD OR OTHER COMPOUNDS HARMFUL IF SWALLOWED. Do not apply on any interior surfaces of a dwelling or of a place used for the care of children or on window sills, toys, cribs or other furniture which might be chewed by children. Wash thoroughly after handling and before eating or smoking. Close container after each use. KEEP OUT OF REACH OF CHILDREN"

Enforcement of the act was given to the Commissioner of Consumer Protection. He has the power to seize paint packaged, distributed, sold or offered for sale in violation of the act. But an attempt to put meaningful fines into the penalties provisions of both the 1967 and 1969 laws was thwarted by a last minute compromise engineered in the Legislature at the behest of interests sympathetic to the paint retailing industry.

Thus, on the books today, it is illegal to sell paint with hazardous concentrations of lead unless prominent warning labels are on the cans; it is illegal to use lead paints in the interiors of any public housing projects; it is illegal to use such paint in apartment houses of three or more units; and the State has restricted its purchases of lead paints to a few intense colors apparently requiring lead salts. Yet, the menace of lead poisoning has not been conquered.

In part, the 1971 legislative package drawn up by the Governor's Lead Task Force, upon which I was privileged to serve, is directed to further the enforcement of this existing legislative framework. In part, the proposed bills attempt to attack the underlying causes of lead poisoning, the coats of lead paints in our existing housing stock accumulated over many decades of neglect.

Thus, one bill will require each doctor, hospital or laboratory to report within 48 hours to the State Commissioner of Health and to the local

Health Director, the name and address of "each person found or suspected to have a level of lead in the blood equal to or greater than .04 milligrams per 100 grams of blood or any other abnormal body burden of lead." This bill gives immunity to the doctor or institution so reporting. Most important, the bill requires the local Director of Health to "make or cause to be made an epidemiological investigation of the source of the lead" and to report the investigation to the local building official who "shall thereupon require such action to be taken . . . as may be necessary to prevent further exposure", including relocation of the family. Within 30 days, the local Health Director must report to the Commissioner on his investigation and the actions taken.

This bill, if enacted, can provide the state-wide statistics necessary for understanding the full impact of lead poisoning. But, most of all, it will put the public spotlight upon those municipalities which do little or nothing in the face of lead poisoning cases by giving concerned local doctors, community groups and politicians hard data. For health directors in such towns will have been required to report to the Commissioner that they simply did nothing to investigate the source of lead poisoning or to prevent further exposure if such were the case.

A second bill aiming at facilitated enforcement of existing legislation is one calling for a $40,000 appropriation to the State Health Department to increase staff and laboratory facilities for performing lead screening and diagnostic tests and studying new methods of lead level detection and related matters. Another such bill would create a nine member watchdog Citizens Advisory Committee on Lead Poisoning to study the operation and enforcement of statutory and housing code provisions, to review reported incidents of lead poisoning and to make recommendations to State and local health departments and to the General Assembly. This latter proposal would, in effect, continue the work of the Governor's Lead Task Force during the next two years.

A fourth measure to assist operation of the existing legislative machinery calls for creation of housing divisions in the Circuit Courts "where needed in Circuits serving urban areas . . . with especially assigned judges and prosecutors with jurisdiction over (1) housing code violation prosecution; (2) summary process action; (3) actions under the Tenant's Representative Act and (4) applications by the Commission on Human Rights for injunctions in housing discrimination cases." The Task Force felt it essential that these provisions be included in any court reorganization legislation that may emerge from the 1971 General Assembly.

Recognizing the need to break radically the cruel circle of poverty and bad housing that characterize lead poisoning incidents, the Task Force proposes a new grant program for State Aid to municipalities (1) to assist them in developing and executing local programs to detect and treat incidents of lead poisoning; and (2) to assist them in developing and executing programs to identify high risk neighborhoods and eliminate the hazards. This bill would assist those localities interested enough to apply by paying up to 75% of the proposed local program costs. The State Health Commissioner would have discretion to allocate the grants according to the dual thrust of the bill—detection and treatment; identification, rehabilitation and preventive maintenance of high risk leaded housing. The Task Force is requesting $500,000 for the biennium for these grants, cognizant of Connecticut's fiscal woes but even more concerned that, without funding and the sense of urgency at the local level that such funds can sustain, more years will pass marked only by more deaths and illnesses among the very children who are most deprived of the amenities and benefits of life in Connecticut's cities.

Another bill aimed at the existing housing stock is an act to enable municipalities to adopt local certificate of occupancy ordinances. Such a local ordinance would apply to any tenement house (three or more units), and deny landlords collection of rent for any period an apartment is occupied, after a vacancy and before a certificate of occupancy has been issued. The certificate would not issue unless the apartment conformed to local housing codes and contained no paint on accessible surfaces with poisonous lead concentrations.

A third such bill would amend existing statutes such as the Fair Rent Commission Law, Tenants Representative Law and the Covenant of Habitability Act to recognize toxic lead base paints as a public health danger and nuisance within the meaning of those housing laws and to give access to relief under their provisions to the tenants affected.

The latter two bills point up a dilemma: to the extent that certificates of occupancy are required and housing codes rigorously enforced, housing is eliminated from the market, rents driven up and overcrowding intensified in the urban core. On the other hand, when housing codes are not enforced, more units may be available but lead poisoning cases multiply. For this reason the Task Force strongly endorsed legislation to accelerate development of new housing throughout the State at rents low and moderate income families can afford. In the words of the Housing Subcommittee Report:

"There is a critical need for new income housing in the State. . . . we cannot eliminate slums unless we construct new housing for low income groups and demolish old housing as soon as it has been vacated. We therefore strongly recommend that legislation be enacted to provide all communities with adequate funding for the construction of new low income housing."

At the same time the Task Force recommended adoption of a state-wide housing code with mandatory minimum standards for all municipalities, modeled after the 1969 American Public Health Association—United States Public Health Service Model Code, but with appropriate reference to the hazards of lead base paints. In this way all 169 Connecticut towns would be required to protect against dangerous peeling, flaking lead base paints in dwellings.

These nine legislative topics were not intended by the Task Force to represent an exhaustive list of possible legislation. Nor would enactment of the suggested bills be a panacea. The hard work must be done at the local enforcement level if the scourge of lead poisoning in young children is ever to be overcome.

Other measures, although not specifically endorsed by the Governor's Lead Task Force, which could be helpful in the fight against lead poisoning, include enactment of a Child Protection and Toy Safety Act for Connecticut, restoration of appropriate fines for violations of Public Acts 533 and 743 (the 1969 and 1967 Lead Paint Statutes) and adequate appropriations for the Connecticut Research Commission. Thus, the former could give the Commissioner of Consumer Protection power to ban from intrastate sales in Connecticut toys and household substances so hazardous that warning labels alone are not sufficient safeguards; such a Child Protection and Toy Safety Act should encompass toys and household substances painted with poisonous lead base paints. Of course, restoration of appropriate penalties for violation of the existing Lead Paint Statutes would facilitate enforcement of those acts. And adequate appropriations at the disposal of the Connecticut Research Commission for grant allocations would enable research grants to be made to those engaged in research in the field of lead poisoning—should timely application be made.

Finally, dealing sensibly with the childhood disease of lead poisoning points up the imperative need to rationalize the delivery of health care services in Connecticut. The 1971 session will face the continuing dramatic rise in hospital and medical costs. Hopefully, one of the means not only for combating these steeply rising costs, but also for providing adequate health care for the kinds of families in which lead poisoning takes a toll would be the encouragement of community group health plans and centers.

Ultimately, the threat of lead poisoning will remain with us in Connecticut until our constricted and unbalanced housing market is opened up. Until the suburban noose around the center cities is broken, until there is freedom of access to decent housing for all families at reasonable costs, poor families with young children will continue to live in core cities in dilapidated housing surrounded by hazardous concentration of lead lurking in peeling, flaking paint on walls and window sills, doors and railings. This basic and tragic malady the 1971 session of the Connecticut General Assembly will doubtless not solve. Perhaps, with the support of the medical profession and others engaged in health and housing, a real start can be made.

Lead In Human And Animal Tissues

NATURALLY OCCURRING CONCENTRATIONS OF ALPHA-EMITTING ISOTOPES IN A NEW ENGLAND POPULATION

VILMA R. HUNT , EDWARD P. RADFORD Jr. and ASCHER SEGALL

INTRODUCTION

THIS REPORT is part of a larger epidemiological study, which was done at the Harvard School of Public Health on the relation of natural low-level radiation exposure to human disease.[1] The natural radioactivity of the environment was estimated through a radiogeological survey of bedrock radioactivity in Maine, New Hampshire and Vermont,[2] a personnel-monitoring survey of population exposure to external gamma radiation in selected areas of high and low bedrock radioactivity, and a survey of the concentration of alpha-emitting radionuclides in teeth extracted from residents who lived in these areas. The purpose of the latter survey was to estimate the skeletal dose rate from naturally-occurring bone-seeking radioelements in order to determine whether sources in the immediate environment might influence this kind of background exposure.

A radiochemical method for the analysis of a single tooth for radium-226, radium-224 (daughter of the longer lived parents radium-228, half-life 5.8 yr and thorium-228, half-life 1.9 yr) and polonium-210 (daughter of lead-210, half-life 21.4 yr) was developed,[3] and an evaluation of the suitability of teeth as indicators of the skeletal burden of alpha-emitting elements was made.[4] Our conclusion was that teeth from individuals of known residence history were adequate for comparison of skeletal levels of alpha-emitting elements in different human populations. Recently this conclusion has been substantiated by LOVAAS and HURSH[5] in a study involving a larger number of bone types. The intercommunity comparisons for eight different geological regions have already been reported,[1] and no correlation of background exposure to place of residence was demonstrated. This paper will present a more detailed account of the results obtained from the analyses of teeth.

MATERIALS AND METHODS

Dentists throughout Vermont and New Hampshire collected the teeth. A special packet was supplied for each patient, so that the name, age, sex, place of birth and length of residence in the town could be noted at the time of extraction. The teeth were dried and sealed in the packet for forwarding to our laboratory. From the large number of teeth sent to us we were able to fulfil a number of requirements: (a) lifetime residence of the donor in a particular locality, though in a few cases of elderly persons a residence time of more than 40 yr was acceptable; (b) relatively little caries, with minimal volume of filling amalgam; (c) approximate matching by age and sex between the Vermont and New Hampshire communities.

The teeth were prepared by removing any filling material with a dental drill. Calculus and dentin discolored by dental caries or amalgam fillings were also removed. Note was taken of the class of tooth and the approximate fraction of the crown of the tooth which remained after preparation. The total sample was a random assortment of permanent incisors, canines, premolars and molars.

In the radiochemical technique used for analysis, polonium-210, radium-226 and radium-224 were all determined on a single tooth.[3] After the tooth was dissolved in concentrated hydrochloric acid, polonium-210 was first plated from the tooth solution on to a silver disc by electro-chemical displacement. The supernatant was then available for radium separation by a co-precipitation method modified from that of GOLDIN.[6] Radium-226 was determined in equilibrium with its short-lived daughters. The method of analysis of radium-224 in the presence of radium-226 has been presented in detail elsewhere.[3] In this report we have assumed radium-224 to be in equilibrium with its parent thorium-228 (half-life 1.9 yr). However, the equilibrium state of thorium-228 with its parent radium-228 is uncertain,[7] both in vivo before extraction of the teeth and for the subsequent period until analysis. Although PETROW and coworkers have argued that thorium-228 should not be used as an indicator of radium-228 levels, their evidence applies to plants and short-lived bone tissues.[7] The only teeth analyzed by these authors were two bovine samples, which showed values of radium-228 and thorium-228 close to equilibrium. For this reason we have taken radium-224 to be a measure of radium-228 in correcting for

the decay subsequent to extraction of the teeth. If thorium-228 actually were unsupported by radium-228 this assumption would underestimate the amount of thorium-228 which was present at the time of extraction. Between the above two possibilities, the differences in calculated doses to the calcified tissues are not great because of the small amount of activity from this chain.

Due to the one to three year period which elapsed from the time of extraction until analysis, polonium-210 (half-life 138.4 days) could be assumed to be in equilibrium with its parent lead-210 (half-life 21.4 yr). Our results therefore, are reported as lead-210, radium-226 and radium-228 in picocuries per gram ash (pCi/g ash). All results for lead-210 and radium-228 have been corrected to the time of collection (average time 2 yr). For the average amounts of activity measured, the coefficients of variation of the individual radiochemical determinations were about 10% for polonium-210, 12% for radium-226 and 25% for radium-224, when the planchets were counted for 48 hr. Longer counting times were sometimes required for samples very low in activity.[3] Ash content was calculated from the calcium determination,[8] on the basis that the ratio of total ash to calcium is 2.6.[9]

RESULTS

Table 1 shows the concentration of lead-210 and radium-226 by sex and age in decades in New Hampshire and Vermont. For radium-228, results in a sample of 55 teeth are given in Table 2 by decade of age. There were too few analyses to make a comparison for this isotope between New Hampshire and Vermont with subdivisions by sex and age.

Table 3 shows the concentrations of lead-210 and radium-226 in 160 teeth from eight localities in Vermont and New Hampshire of different geological character.[1] Radium-228 values are also shown for 55 of these teeth. The four New Hampshire communities are in the vicinity of igneous bedrock, while the four Vermont communities are located in an area of sedimentary bedrock. The mean values for New Hampshire and Vermont are shown in this table for which data from both males and females were combined. Small differences are

Table 1. *Concentrations of lead-210, radium-226 by sex and age in decades, New Hampshire and Vermont**

	New Hampshire Lead-210 pCi/g ash ± S.E. of mean		Radium-226 pCi/g ash ± S.E. of mean	
	Female	Male	Female	Male
0–9	0.048 ± 0.012 (4)	0.057 ± 0.040 (2)	0.008 ± 0.002 (4)	0.013 ± (2)
10–19	0.054 ± 0.003 (13)	0.042 ± 0.007 (9)	0.019 ± 0.003 (13)	0.016 ± 0.003 (9)
20–29	0.050 ± 0.008 (10)	0.072 ± 0.010 (12)	0.026 ± 0.007 (10)	0.014 ± 0.002 (11)
30–39	0.066 ± 0.011 (8)	0.064 ± 0.006 (9)	0.019 ± 0.002 (8)	0.015 ± 0.003 (9)
40–49	0.064 ± 0.010 (10)	0.073 ± 0.009 (7)†	0.023 ± 0.004 (10)	0.017 ± 0.003 (8)
50–59	0.066 ± 0.020 (4)	0.078 ± 0.008 (8)	0.017 ± 0.004 (4)	0.028 ± 0.010 (8)
60–69	0.051 ± 0.008 (5)	0.089 ± 0.019 (3)	0.031 ± 0.009 (5)	0.021 ± 0.004 (3)
>70	0.041 ± 0.013 (3)	0.064 ± 0.014 (6)	0.021 ± 0.003 (3)	0.022 ± 0.007 (6)
Pooled mean	0.056 ± 0.004 (57)	0.066 ± 0.004 (56)	0.021 ± 0.002 (57)	0.018 ± 0.002 (56)
	Vermont			
0–9	0.058 (1)	0.050 (2)	0.005 (1)	0.007 (2)
10–19	0.044 ± 0.004 (12)	0.060 ± 0.005 (11)	0.009 ± 0.001 (12)	0.020 ± 0.006 (11)
20–29	0.055 ± 0.004 (15)	0.072 ± 0.013 (9)	0.014 ± 0.002 (15)	0.010 ± 0.003 (9)
30–39	0.044 ± 0.008 (6)	0.068 ± 0.007 (7)	0.009 ± 0.002 (6)	0.010 ± 0.002 (7)
40–49	0.065 ± 0.011 (5)	0.057 ± 0.007 (9)	0.011 ± 0.002 (5)	0.013 ± 0.004 (9)
50–59	0.061 ± 0.007 (7)	0.051 ± 0.003 (6)	0.017 ± 0.005 (7)	0.013 ± 0.003 (6)
60–69	0.043 ± 0.004 (3)	0.071 ± 0.007 (5)	0.014 ± 0.005 (3)	0.013 ± 0.003 (5)
>70	0.032 ± 0.002 (2)*	0.040 ± 0.009 (4)	0.021 ± 0.007 (3)	0.013 ± 0.005 (4)
Pooled mean	0.051 ± 0.003 (51)	0.061 ± 0.003 (53)	0.013 ± 0.001 (52)	0.013 ± 0.001 (53)

* Numbers in parentheses indicate number of teeth analyzed.
† One extreme value omitted.

present but when detailed statistical analyses were made only the radium-226 difference was found to be statistically significant ($p < 0.05$). Analyses of variance of the male and female samples of lead-210 and radium-226 in the

Table 2. *Concentrations of radium-228 by age in decades**

	pCi/g ash ± S.E. of mean
0–9	0.010 ± 0.002 (3)
10–19	0.011 ± 0.002 (10)
20–29	0.009 ± 0.002 (11)
30–39	0.006 ± 0.002 (9)
40–49	0.004 ± 0.001 (12)
50–59	0.007 ± 0.003 (4)
60–69	0.007 ± 0.006 (2)
<70	0.010 ± 0.002 (4)
Pooled mean	0.008 ± 0.003 (55)

* Numbers in parentheses indicate number of teeth analyzed.

eight communities indicated that only radium-226 in the males showed significant variation between communities ($p < 0.05$). The male and female samples for radium-228 were combined and showed no significant regional variation.

Additional teeth from New Hampshire and Vermont had been analyzed during this study and have been included in the following results and in Table 1.

Lead-210

Figure 1 shows the wide range of values obtained for lead-210 in a sample of 219 teeth, 0.009 pCi/g ash to 2.237 pCi/g ash. The mean was 0.070 pCi/g ash, the median was 0.057 pCi/g ash and the interquartile range was 0.041 pCi/g ash to 0.720 pCi/g ash. This markedly skewed distribution was particularly affected by two individuals, one with a value of 0.385 pCi/g ash and the other with a value

New Hampshire	²¹⁰Pb pCi/g ash ± S.E. of mean	²²²Ra pCi/g ash ± S.E. of mean	²²⁸Ra pCi/g ash ± S.E. of mean
Concord	0.054 ± 0.007 (20)	0.014 ± 0.002 (20)	0.005 ± 0.001 (11)
Conway	0.064 ± 0.007 (20)	0.025 ± 0.005 (20)	0.003 ± 0.001 (3)
Franklin	0.066 ± 0.006 (20)	0.016 ± 0.002 (20)	0.006 ± 0.002 (8)
Manchester	0.060 ± 0.006 (20)	0.019 ± 0.004 (20)	0.010 ± 0.001 (9)
Mean	0.061 ± 0.003	0.018 ± 0.002	0.006 ± 0.001
Vermont			
Bennington	0.056 ± 0.006 (20)	0.009 ± 0.001 (20)	0.010 ± 0.003 (4)
Burlington	0.050 ± 0.005 (20)	0.010 ± 0.002 (20)	0.010 ± 0.002 (11)
Middlebury	0.061 ± 0.005 (15)	0.020 ± 0.005 (15)	0.005 (2)
Rutland	0.054 ± 0.003 (25)	0.014 ± 0.002 (25)	0.009 ± 0.002 (7)
Mean	0.055 ± 0.002	0.013 ± 0.001	0.009 ± 0.002
Significance of difference N.H. vs. Vermont	N.S.	$p < 0.05$	N.S.

* Numbers in parentheses indicate number of teeth analysed.

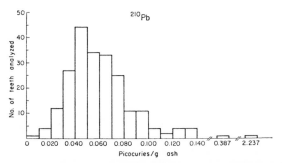

²¹⁰Pb

FIG. 1. Frequency distribution of lead-210 content in 219 teeth from individuals living in northern New England. Note that abscissa is broken to show two very high measurements in two individuals.

of 2.237 pCi/g ash. In the latter extreme case we attempted to obtain a medical history. The tooth had been extracted from a 74-yr-old woman who lived in Brandon, Vermont. She reported that she had been hospitalized for tuberculosis about 1914, but did not remember details of the medication she received. No smoking history was obtained. There was no evidence of high levels of radioactivity in the water supply. The radium-226 value for her tooth was 0.037 pCi/g ash. We can give no explanation for the high lead-210 value, nor was there any likelihood of contamination during analysis, as other teeth analyzed on the same day were not remarkable. The mean value ± standard error for the concentration of lead-210 in females was 0.054 ± 0.002 pCi/g ash and 0.064 ± 0.003 pCi/g ash for males. The aforementioned extreme values were excluded for this analysis. The difference was

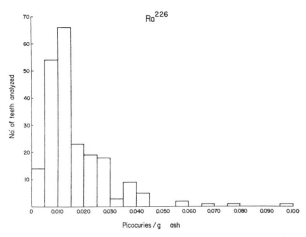

Fig. 2. Frequency distribution of radium-226 content in 218 teeth from individuals living in northern New England.

statistically significant $(t = 2.74; \; p < 0.01)$. The concentration of lead-210 in teeth was not significantly correlated with age in either sex, or in the total sample.

Radium-226

Figure 2 shows the distribution of radium-226 in 218 teeth. The range of radium-226 values was not as wide as that found for lead-210; 0.001 pCi/g ash to 0.097 pCi/g ash, with the interquartile range from 0.008 pCi/g ash to 0.021 pCi/g ash. The mean value was 0.016 pCi/g ash and the median value was 0.012 pCi/g ash. There was no sex difference in the concentration of this isotope in teeth. The radium-226 concentration tends to increase slightly with age though there was no significant sex difference in the correlation. For the correlation with age, when both sexes were combined, r was $+0.165$ $(p < 0.01)$.

Radium-228

Radium-228 values range from zero to 0.021 pCi/g ash. There were 7 teeth from towns in New Hampshire, in which radium-228 was not detected. The limit of detectability was 0.002 pCi/g ash. The interquartile range

was 0.004–0.011 pCi/g ash, the mean value was 0.008 pCi/g ash and the median value was 0.007 pCi/g ash. There was no significant sex difference in the concentration of this isotope, nor was there a significant sex difference in the decline of concentration with age. However, when the male and female samples were combined there was a small negative correlation with age $(r = -0.30)$ $(p < 0.05)$.

Computation of the lead-210 to radium-226 ratios in individual teeth gave values of 1–60 times, in part a reflection of the wide range of values found for lead-210 and radium-226 content. There was no correlation between the amounts of lead-210 and radium-226 found in a single tooth. Ratios of radium-228 to radium-226 were also variable and ranged from 0 to 3, most samples having a ratio well below 1.

DISCUSSION

We have previously discussed the suitability of measuring the concentrations of alpha-emitting isotopes in teeth for the estimation of radiation dose to the skeleton.[4] This series of analyses has been made to study a certain population, in order to estimate the skeletal dose rate from naturally occurring radioactive

100

elements. The 219 teeth could have been pooled as one large sample to obtain the same estimate, but any evidence of variability within the population would have been lost. The variation in concentrations of the three radio-elements measured was 15-fold or more, which indicates that retention in teeth may not be solely dependent on amounts being ingested from food, water and air, inasmuch as in a population of stable residence in Vermont and New Hampshire one would expect relatively constant ingestion rates for different individuals. Other biological factors such as absorption by the gut, or retention, translocation and excretion from the body probably make more contribution to individual variation in this population than differences in ingestion. These factors are as yet poorly understood, particularly for low levels of ingested radioelements. Lead-210 metabolism may be reasonably related to other lead isotopes, which would indicate that lead uptake and storage may be quite variable in the general population. One source of lead-210 is very probably cigarette smoke. HOLTZMAN and ILCEWICZ[10] have shown that concentration of lead-210 in rib bones of cigarette smokers is about twice that of non-smokers. Unfortunately, smoking histories were not obtained at the time the teeth used in this sample were collected so that comparisons could not be made between smokers and non-smokers in the present study.

The purpose of our measurements was to determine whether local differences in bedrock composition would be reflected in skeletal burdens of radium isotopes and their daughters. There was little evidence of a difference associated with different places of residence, where igneous or sedimentary rocks were the chief bedrock types. A slightly increased amount of radium-226 was found in New Hampshire residents living in an area where igneous rocks might be expected to contribute some radium to local food or water.

We found no age trend in the lead-210 content of teeth. Tooth enamel undergoes no remodelling after formation and there is a minimum of ion exchange.[11] Dentine probably contains higher concentrations than enamel due to higher diffusion rates of tissue fluids and ion exchange.[4] There have been no reports of marked increases with age in the concentration of lead-210 and radium in the human skeleton, though there may be a slight increase found in trabecular bone.[12] In the case of radium-228 there was a very small negative correlation with age ($r = -0.30$, $p < 0.05$), which may be attributable to the short half-life of 5.8 yr for this radioelement. Radium-226 concentrations showed a small positive correlation with age, ($r = +0.165$, $p < 0.01$).

For the purposes of this survey, we have made the assumption that the skeletal tissues are in equilibrium with the environment, to the extent that our data do not indicate a marked retention of these radioelements with age. We are assuming that the concentrations of radioelements found represent a measure of the radioactive elements retained by the skeleton in the population under study.

We have compared the results reported in this study with those from earlier reports in Table 4. The concentrations of lead-210 and radium-226 are in general agreement, though a wider range of values is apparent in the present study, probably due to the larger sample size.

The concentrations found in these teeth may be used to estimate skeletal doses delivered by alpha-emitters to bone marrow or osteocytes. We have assumed that lead-210 in spongy bone is twice the concentration in teeth.[4] LOVAAS and HURSH[5] found slightly lower ratios comparing femoral head and rib teeth and we agree that the variation in this ratio is high. Because of the individual variation observed within the group, an average figure for bone dose is intended simply to indicate the importance of these elements relative to other background sources. Similarly because the distribution of these elements within a single bone is not uniform, a single dose factor is not likely to apply. For example, we have found that trabecular bone may contain up to ten times the average amount of all three elements present in the whole bone.[4] Nevertheless, it is instructive to obtain approximate estimates.

By modification of the equation of SPIERS and BURCH,[19] we may express the average dose rate D, in mrad/yr:

$$D = 5CE\bar{F}$$

where C is the isotope concentration in pCi/g

Table 4. *Comparison of results with earlier studies*

Reference	Year	Mean	Range	Sample size	Locality
		Lead-210 pCi/g ash of bone			
This report		0.137*			
		0.118†	0.018–4.474	219	Northeast U.S.A.
10	1966	0.135‡	0.071–0.172	6	Midwest U.S.A.
10	1966	0.285§	0.179–0.502	13	Midwest U.S.A.
12	1963	0.146	0.037–0.454	128	Midwest U.S.A.
4	1963	0.142	0.035–0.320	25	Northeast U.S.A.
13	1960	0.169	0.018–1.330	45	Midwest U.S.A.
		Radium-226 pCi/g ash of bone			
This report		0.016	0.001–0.097	218	Northeast U.S.A.
4	1963	0.014	0.002–0.045	25	Northeast U.S.A.
13	1960	0.037	0.010–0.191	45	Midwest U.S.A.
14	1960		0.016–0.070	6	
15	1960	0.012	0.005–0.027	42	Midwest U.S.A.
16	1959	0.008	0.003–0.030	140	Northeast U.S.A.
17	1958	0.016	0.006–0.050	50	Northwest U.S.A.
18	1950	0.050	0.019–0.090	20	Northeast U.S.A.

* Lead-210 in bone is twice the concentration in teeth.
† Two extreme values omitted
‡ Non-smokers
§ Smokers

bone ash, E is the alpha energy in MeV released per initial decay, including the retained short-lived daughters, and $\bar{F}$ is the geometrical factor, dependent primarily on whether lacunae, Haversian canals or bone marrow adjacent to bone are being considered.

Spiers and Burch's formula is:

$$D(\text{rad/week}) = 240C\Sigma(nE)\bar{F}$$

where C is given in uCi/g wet bone. The equation we have used gives the dose in mrad/yr, and the isotope concentration in pCi/g ash, with $\Sigma(nE)$ and $\bar{F}$ the same as Spiers and Burch. To convert μCi/g wet bone to pCi/gm bone ash, the conversion factor is 0.4×10^{-6} μCi/g wet bone per pCi/g bone ash, on the assumption that bone ash is 40% of wet bone weight. Therefore, the constant 240 in Spiers and Burch's formula becomes $240 \times 52{,}000$ mrad/yr per rad/week $\times 0.4 \times 10^{-6} \simeq 5.0$.

To determine the energy E we have assumed that radon-222 is 30% retained from radium-226

decay in bone, radium-224 is 50% of thorium-228 and radium-228 in bone,[20] and polonium-210 is in equilibrium with lead-210 in bone.[12] Table 5 gives results of these calculations. Also, in Table 5 the rad dose has been converted to rem by use of a quality factor of 10.[21]

We may compare the doses calculated in Table 5 with a dose from other radiation sources of about 140 mrem/yr (approximately 60 from cosmic rays, including neutrons, 60 from external gamma exposure and 20 from internal beta and gamma-ray sources, primarily potassium-40). It is clear that the alpha doses calculated in Table 5 are far from negligible, especially from polonium-210, the alpha emitting daughter of lead-210. For this isotope a soft tissue component may also be present, and therefore its contribution in bone may be even greater than indicated in Table 3. It is also clear that polonium-210 is the major background source of alpha radiation even in bone tissue where radium-226 and radium-228 are concentrated. This conclusion is in agreement with observations of others.[12,22]

Table 5. Estimated background dose to spongy bone tissues from radium-226, radium-228 and lead-210 from data in this report. Concentrations of radium-226 and radium-228 in teeth assumed to be characteristic of bone. Concentrations of lead-210 in teeth assumed to be 0.5 that in bone.[4] *Alpha radiation dose only*

A

Osteocytes in 10μ lacuna or Haversian canal

$\bar{F} = 1.35$

	C pCi/g ash	E MeV	D mrad/yr	Dose (QF − 10) mrem/yr
Radium-226	0.016	10.6	1.15	11.5
Radium-228	0.008	18.7	1.01	10.1
Lead-210	0.118*	5.3	4.23	42.3
			Total	63.9

B

Bone marrow cells within 10μ of bone

$\bar{F} = 0.66$

Radium-226	0.016	10.6	0.56	5.6
Radium-228	0.008	18.7	0.49	4.9
Lead-210	0.118*	5.3	2.06	20.6
			Total	31.1

* Mean excludes two extreme values.

There is a significant difference between males and females in the concentration of lead-210. A sex difference in the metabolism of lead may be possible, but it seems that occupational exposure and smoking habits would be a more likely explanation. In the mixed population presented in this study, of unknown smoking history, it is reasonable to assume that a sex difference in the degree of smoking might be reflected in the dissimilar concentrations of lead-210 in the skeleton. From our data it can be calculated that the males in this population experience a 10% higher background radiation dose to the osteocytes and bone marrow cells from the naturally occurring alpha-emitting radioelements than do females.

SUMMARY AND CONCLUSIONS

Teeth from people living in several communities in Vermont and New Hampshire were analyzed radiochemically for radium-226, radium-224 (as a measure of the parents thorium-228 and radium-228) and polonium-210 (as a measure of lead-210), in order to determine whether differences in bedrock radioactivity in the area of these communities could be related to differences in burdens of alpha-emitting elements in calcified tissues. The only statistical difference observed was a slight increase in radium-226 levels in New Hampshire when compared with Vermont ($p < 0.05$). The mean values for radium-226, radium-228 and lead-210 expressed as pCi/g ash were 0.016, 0.008 and 0.070, respectively. The distributions were highly skewed, and in a few individuals much higher concentrations were found, although no explanation for these unusual results was available.

There was no age trend observed for lead-210 concentrations, a very small positive correlation of age with radium-226 concentration and a very small negative correlation of age with radium-228 concentration. Our hypothesis is that the concentrations observed depended on relative equilibrium with the environment. Lead-210 concentration in males was significantly higher than in females. Lead-210 and its alpha-emitting daughter, polonium-210 are present in much higher concentrations than radium-226, and in this population polonium-210 is more significant as a source of background alpha radiation exposure than radium-226 or radium-228, even in calcified tissues where the latter are concentrated.

Acknowledgements—We are greatly indebted to DWYN SHERRY and VIRGINIA GILMORE for the analytical work. This study would not have been possible without the enthusiastic cooperation of the Dental Societies of Vermont and New Hampshire, and to the many individual dentists who so carefully provided us with suitable specimens. We take great pleasure in acknowledging their contribution.

The study was supported by Research Grant No. 6715, National Institutes of Health, United States Public Health Service, and by the Higgens Fund, Harvard University, and the Radcliffe Institute for Independent Study, Radcliffe College.

REFERENCES

1. A. SEGALL, *Science* **140**, 1337 (1963).
2. M. P. BILLINGS, unpublished data.

3. E. P. RADFORD, JR., V. R. HUNT and D. SHERRY, *Radiat. Res.* **19,** 298 (1963).
4. V. R. HUNT, E. P. RADFORD, JR. and A. J. SEGALL, *Int. J. Radiat. Biol.* **7,** 277 (1963).
5. A. I. LOVAAS and J. B. HURSH, *Health Phys.* **14,** 549 (1968).
6. A. S. GOLDIN, *Analyt. Chem.* **33,** 406 (1961).
7. H. G. PETROW, A. COVER, W. SCHIESSLE and E. PARSONS, *Analyt. Chem.* **36,** 1600 (1964).
8. R. G. YALMAN, W. BRUEGEMANN, P. T. BAKER and S. M. GARN, *Analyt. Chem.* **31,** 1230 (1959).
9. W. S. SPECTOR, (Editor) *Handbook of Biological Data*, p. 73. W. B. Saunders, Philadelphia (1956).
10. R. B. HOLTZMAN and F. H. ILCEWICZ, *Science* **153,** 1259 (1966).
11. W. F. NEUMAN and M. W. NEUMAN, *The Chemical Dynamics of Bone Mineral.* University of Chicago Press, Chicago (1958).
12. R. B. HOLTZMAN, *Health Phys.* **9,** 385 (1963).
13. R. B. HOLTZMAN, Argonne National Laboratory 6199 (1960).
14. A. F. STEHNEY, *A Symposium on Radioisotopes in the Biosphere* (Edited by R. S. Caldecott and L. A. SNYDER). University of Minnesota Press (1960).
15. H. F. LUCAS JR., Argonne National Laboratory 6297 (1960).
16. A. WALTON, R. KOLOGRIVOV and J. L. KULP, *Health Phys.* **1,** 409 (1959).
17. R. F. PALMER and F. B. QUEEN, *Am. J. Roentg.* **79,** 521 (1958).
18. J. B. HURSH and A. A. GATES, *Nucleonics* **7,** 46 (1950).
19. F. W. SPIERS and P. R. H. BURCH, *Adv. Biol. Med. Phys.* **5,** 425 (1957).
20. Report of the R.B.E. Committee to the International Commissions on Radiological Protection and on Radiological Units and Measurements, *Health Phys.* **9,** 357 (1963).
21. Report of ICRP on Permissible Dose for Internal Radiation (1959), *Health Phys.* **3,** 1 (1960).
22. C. R. HILL, *Nature, Lond.* **208,** 423 (1965).

CONCENTRATIONS OF ^{210}Po, ^{226}Ra AND ^{228}Th IN THE CHOROID OF THE EYE, PARTICULARLY IN CATTLE

V. R. HUNT

INTRODUCTION

THE naturally occurring alpha-emitting isotopes, radium and ^{210}Po are normally present in animal and human tissues, especially the skeleton (Radford *et al.*, 1964; Di Ferrante, 1964).

Rehfeld *et al.* (1960) reported pathologic changes in the eyes of beagle dogs after intravenous injection of high concentrations of ^{226}Ra. They also found that ^{226}Ra accumulated in the pigmented parts of the eye. The Atlas of Erleksova (1960) shows an autoradiograph of a sagittal section of the eyeball of a dog; the radioactivity is due to injected ^{210}Po. It appears to be concentrated in the choroid and iris.

In cattle, squamous cell carcinoma of the eye is the most common form of neoplastic disease (Russell, 1956).

From this evidence it seemed worthwhile to analyse pigmented tissues of the eye of cattle for the naturally occurring radioelements, radium and ^{210}Po, in order to find if concentration of these elements did in fact occur. They are present in food and water supplies throughout the world, and vary considerably in concentration. This variation is dependent in part on the geological characteristics of the places of origin.

METHODS

Eyes were obtained from cattle, by gross dissection of the orbital contents after slaughter at the abattoir. A total of 33 bovine eyes were analysed, 12 from an area 30 miles west of Boston (Eastern United States), 10 supplied by a Minneapolis (Midwest United States) abattoir, and 12 from a supplier of biological research material. The latter series of eyes had been obtained from an abattoir in Minneapolis in the midwest of the United States 4 months before our analyses and were preserved in formalin. The eyes from Boston and Minneapolis were fresh frozen and analysed (after thawing) within 2–3 weeks of death.

The cornea, retina, choroid, iris and sclera could all be easily separated (Fig. 1). In some cases the retina was somewhat contaminated by pigment grains, which escaped from the adjacent choroid. The tapetum lucidum was included with the choroid.

The methods used for separating radium and ^{210}Po have been described elsewhere (Radford *et al.*, 1964) and will be briefly outlined here. The sample is wet ashed with hot concentrated hydrochloric acid, polonium is plated on silver, and the radium isotopes are then co-precipitated with $PbSO_4$ and $BaSO_4$. We obtain 100 % recovery of ^{210}Po and 70 % recovery of ^{226}Ra added to tissue during digestion. Radium and ^{210}Po samples are counted in gas flow proportional counters with background alpha counts in the range of 0·5–1·0 counts per hour. ^{224}Ra content is calculated from grow-in data

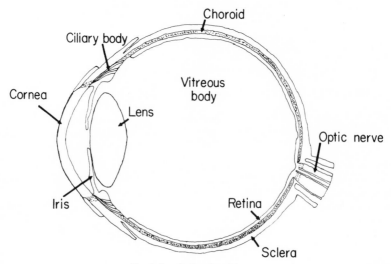

Choroid

Ciliary body

Cornea

Vitreous
body

Lens

Optic nerve

Iris

Retina

Sclera

FIG. 1. A sagittal section of the eye.

derived from successive radium counts. It is reported as ^{228}Th with which ^{224}Ra is in equilibrium due to its short half-life relative to that of the parent.

Results are reported in picocuries per gram wet weight of tissue. It is likely that the wet weights of fresh tissue and that preserved in formalin are not strictly comparable. However, given the limits of the analytical and counting errors of the results, which are approximately 8 % for ^{210}Po, 10 % for ^{226}Ra, and 25 % for ^{228}Th, this possibility has been ignored.

Sixteen analyses were done on the choroid and iris together for ^{210}Po, 15 analyses for ^{226}Ra and 11 for ^{228}Th. The choroid alone was analysed from 17 eyes for ^{210}Po, and ^{226}Ra and from 3 eyes for ^{228}Th. ^{226}Ra and ^{210}Po were measured in the retina for 7 eyes, in the vitreous and aqueous humor for 3 eyes, the cornea for 2 eyes, the sclera for 1 and extraocular muscle for 6 eyes.

RESULTS

The results are shown in Table I. The iris in all cases contained only half to two-thirds the amount of ^{210}Po† per gram wet weight found in the choroid. ^{226}Ra and ^{228}Th values were also lower in the iris. The retina, vitreous and aqueous humor, cornea, sclera and muscle contained only a very small fraction of the amounts of the radioelements found in the choroid and iris. Of these latter eye sections the retina contained the highest concentrations of ^{210}Po, ^{226}Ra and ^{228}Th.

The data from the two geographic regions, Eastern and Midwest United States show considerable differences for all three radioelements. In the Midwest United States the ^{210}Po values are higher and the ^{226}Ra and ^{228}Th values are lower than those in the Eastern United States.

† The present results cannot indicate the equilibrium state of ^{210}Po and its parent ^{210}Pb. The results of further studies are shown in Table III, page 309. Table IV shows results of analyses made on the eyes of several vertebrate species.

Table I. Eastern United States, Boston—fresh

	No. of samples	^{210}Po [a]	^{226}Ra [a]	^{228}Th [a]
Choroid	2	0·367	1·676	0·788
Iris	2	0·234	1·661	0·736
Choroid and iris	10	0·322 ± 0·050	1·159 ± 0·085	0·634 ± 0·098
Retina	1	0·002	0·009	—
Vitreous and aqueous humor	—	—	—	—
Cornea	—	—	—	—
Sclera	—	—	—	—
Muscle	1	0·004	0·017	—

Mid-West United States, Minneapolis—fresh

	No. of samples	^{210}Po [a]	^{226}Ra [a]	^{228}Th [a]
Choroid	8	2·714 ± 0·563	0·740 ± 0·135	0·476 ± 0·027
Iris	8	1·063 ± 0·195	0·354 ± 0·027	—
Choroid and iris	2	0·816	0·134	—
Retina	2	0·341	0·020	—
Vitreous and aqueous humor	2	0·082	0·011	—
Cornea	1	0·025	0·020	—
Sclera	—	—	—	—
Muscle	2	0·024	0·003	—

Mid-West United States, Chicago—formalin preserved

	No. of samples	^{210}Po [a]	^{226}Ra [a]	^{228}Th [a]
Choroid	(7) (7) (5)	1·524 ± 0·299	0·206 ± 0·039	0·322 ± 0·050
Iris	(7) (6) (1)	1·176 ± 0·194	0·122 ± 0·034	0·177
Choroid and iris	(4) (3) (1)	1·153 ± 0·141	0·132 ± 0·028	0·219
Retina	4	0·159	0·018	—
Vitreous and aqueous humor	1	0·024	0·027	—
Cornea	1	0·004	0·012	—
Sclera	1	0·035	0·018	—
Muscle	3	0·006	0·012	—

[a] Expressed as pCi/g wet weight ± standard error of the mean.

DISCUSSION

Radioactivity from ingested radioisotopes is an important contribution to the radiation dose from the environment experienced by animal and man (Dudley, 1959). Usually the concentration of naturally occurring radioelements in animal and human tissues (Table II) is quite low and therefore the design of studies for the detection of possible radiation effects on animal and human populations has been difficult.

We have found relatively high concentrations of ^{226}Ra, ^{228}Th and ^{210}Po in the choroid and the iris of the eyes of cattle. This is in contrast to the low concentrations in the sclera, retina, cornea and

Table II

	^{210}Pb	^{228}Ra	^{228}Th
Man			
Bone (Hunt *et al.*, 1963)	0·018 pCi/g wet wt.	0·014 pCi/g ash	0·009 pCi/g ash
Soft tissue (Little *et al.*, 1964; Lucas, 1960)	0·012 pCi/g wet wt.	0·008 pCi/g ash	—
Cattle			
Bone (Di Ferrante, 1964, Hill *et al.*, 1961)	0·250 pCi/g wet wt.	0·180–2·60pCi/g ash	—
Soft tissue (Table I muscle)	0·011 pCi/g wet wt.	0·011 pCi/g wet wt.	

aqueous and vitreous humor (Table I). These findings indicate that the choroid and iris, which together weigh from 1 to 1·5 g, should be useful in the study of the effects of alpha-emitting radioelements in large animal populations.

The radiation dose to the choroid can be calculated on the basis of the following assumptions.

(a) 1 pCi/g each of ^{210}Po and ^{226}Ra and 0·75 pCi/g of ^{228}Th are present. The distribution throughout the choroid is relatively uniform.

(b) The thickness of the choroid in cattle is 0·16 mm (Prince *et al.*, 1960).

(c) 94·5% of the energy from alpha particles is absorbed in the choroid. The fraction of energy absorbed when the thickness is at least twice the alpha particle range is $1-R/4W$, where R is the average alpha particle range (35 μ) and W is the thickness of the choroid.

(d) ^{222}Rn and daughters are not retained in the choroid due to the 3·8 day half-life of ^{222}Rn, its chemically inert nature and the high vascularity of the choroid.

(e) ^{220}Rn (half-life 54 sec) with its daughter products are 100% retained due to their very short half lives.

(f) The dose from the β emitters in the decay chain has not been included. This would be relatively small when compared with the dose from alpha particles.

(g) A relative biological effectiveness of 10 has been assumed for alpha particles. (Recommendations of the International Commission on Radiological Protection 1955.)

The dose to the choroid under these conditions would be 935 mrem/year from ^{210}Po, 283 mrem/year from ^{226}Ra and 4111 mrem/year from ^{228}Th. The total dose of 5·3 rem/year would be subject to wide variation, aside from possible errors in the assumptions used, which would be dependent, primarily, on geographic differences.

The values for ^{226}Ra in the Boston series are 5 times higher than those for the Midwest preserved series, and 2·5 times the Midwest fresh series. In contrast, ^{210}Po values were by far the highest in the Midwest fresh series, with the Midwest preserved series intermediate and the Boston series only one-eighth those of the highest series. ^{228}Th values in the Boston series were twice those in the Midwest series.

The factors which contribute to such variability are probably the water and food supplies. A wide range of variation for values of ^{226}Ra, ^{228}Th, ^{210}Pb and its daughter ^{210}Po, has been found for treated and untreated water supplies from rivers, wells and springs throughout the United States of America. (Hursh, 1957; Grune *et al.*, 1960; Holtzman, 1964; Lucas *et al.*, 1960). ^{226}Ra has been found in concentrations of 0·017 pCi/l. to 730 pCi/l. ^{210}Pb and ^{210}Po values are generally much lower, with values of 0·2 pCi/l. and 0·016 pCi/l. respectively reported in the Midwest United States. In the same area ^{228}Th concentrations of 8 pCi/l. were found.

High concentrations of ^{210}Pb and ^{210}Po are found in herbage consumed by cattle. (Mayneord *et al.*, 1959; Hill, 1960). An important source of these radioelements is natural fallout, due to the decay of atmospheric ^{222}Rn and its short-lived daughters. Considerable geographic variability in foliar deposition is due to meteorological conditions. Higher concentrations are found in areas of high rainfall. The ^{210}Pb and ^{210}Po content of the soil also contributes to the concentration found in the plant (Tso *et al.*, 1964). Plants grown in soil which contains monazite show higher concentrations of ^{228}Ra and ^{228}Th (Petrow, 1964). Food concentrates are also widely used to feed cattle in the United States. Chapman *et al.* (1963) have estimated a daily consumption of 3255 pCi/day of uranium from this source. It is probable that other radioelements in the uranium chain, at least, would be present also.

Data on the daily food and water intake of dairy cattle are available (Garner, 1963). A 550 kg standard cow consumes daily 8–11 kg of dry matter and drinks 50 l. of water. However, beef cattle are known to consume less.

From these observations it is apparent that the variability of intake of naturally occurring radio-elements could be quite marked, from one region to another, particularly when such large amounts of food and water are consumed each day by cattle.

Another important source of ^{210}Pb and ^{210}Po is from air by the inhalation route (Holtzman, 1965). However, this might be expected to be relatively constant from one continental area to another and certainly not subject to the wide fluctuations which occur in water and food supplies.

Neoplasia is the cause of condemnation in 0·227% of the 25 million beasts slaughtered per year in federally inspected abattoirs (Brandly *et al.*, 1963). Federal inspection is made on approximately two-thirds of the cattle slaughtered in the United States. Of these condemnations 88% are due to squamous cell carcinoma of the eye. The epidemiologic data do not take into account animals which die from the tumor on farms, those which are treated before slaughter nor those slaughtered in non-federally inspected abattoirs. Therefore a good estimate of the prevalence of this carcinoma in the living animal population is not available (Russell *et al.*, 1956). There is considerable regional variation; the highest prevalence in the United States is in the southwest, with a maximum of 10% reported in some herds. The disease has been reported from Europe, South America, Africa, Asia and Australasia.

Squamous cell carcinoma of the eye occurs predominantly in cattle more than 1-year-old and it is rare in other species. Breed groups differ in susceptibility, and the breed contribution to suscepti-bility is related to pigmentation of the bulbar conjunctiva. Excessive sunlight may be a contributing factor (Anderson *et al.*, 1961). White faced Herefords are particularly susceptible. They make up over 90% of the cattle slaughtered for food in the United States. Attempts to find an associated virus have not yet been definitely successful (Sykes *et al.*, 1961).

The squamous cell carcinoma arises from the conjunctiva of the eye at or on either side of the limbus (corneal-scleral junction) (Fig. 2), and less frequently from the conjunctival skin junction of the eyelids. These are areas characterized by embryological junction of epithelial surfaces (Monlux *et al.*, 1957). The lesion first appears as a white firm plaque only a few millimeters in size. It gradually enlarges as a papillary lesion or ulcer, and progresses to carcinoma *in situ* and finally to invasive carcinoma (Steiner *et al.*, 1951). Multiple squamous cell carcinomas occur in single eyes and involvement of both eyes is sometimes found.

Several factors amenable to further study are apparent. The choroid is a small portion of a large mammal. It is available in unlimited quantity as it is not put to any use in the meat industry. It has been found possible to culture eye tissue (Sykes, 1961), so that successive generations of cells can be studied, and, presumably, chromosomes and chromosomal changes. The epithelial cells are especially susceptible to neoplastic change for reasons as yet unknown.

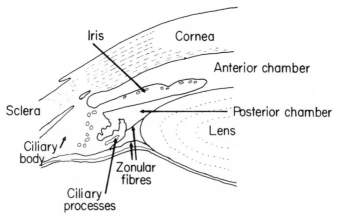

FIG. 2. The limbus of the eye: zone of transition between cornea and sclera.

These factors present opportunities for the study of cell changes with age in herds of pedigreed cattle, of far more homogeneous genetic composition than human groups. The radiation dose can be more accurately defined than is the case with radiation dose to larger organs, such as the skeleton.

Primarily, it would be of interest to learn if the radiation dose to the choroid is a factor in the high prevalence of squamous cell carcinoma of the eye in cattle. Can radiation induced chromosome aberrations be recognized and related to the radiation dose delivered to critical cells in the eye? Are cell-killing effects present at the radiation dose levels found in the eyes of cattle? To what extent are other factors such as inherited susceptibility, environmental hazards and possible viruses enhanced in their carcinogenic role by the presence of such radiation dose levels as have been presented in this report? Cole and Nowell (1965) have recently outlined a conceptual sequence of events in radiation carcinogenesis in an attempt to incorporate many of the complex interactions which appear to operate at the subcellular, cellular and whole animal levels. It may be possible to evaluate some of these factors by further study of the eyes of cattle.

SUMMARY

The iris and choroid of the eye of cattle are shown to contain the naturally occurring radio elements, ^{226}Ra, ^{228}Th, and ^{210}Po, in amounts of about 1 pCi/g wet weight of each of these radio elements. This is not the case with the retina, sclera, cornea, vitreous and aqueous humor.

The possible radiation dose to the choroid is calculated to be about 5·3 rem/year, based on a certain set of assumptions, which are outlined.

The source of the radioelements is primarily from water and food supplies, and to a lesser degree from the air. Geographic variation is apparent.

Squamous cell carcinoma of the eye is a major cause of condemnation of cattle. The neoplasia usually appears on the conjunctiva of the eye in the region of the corneal-scleral junction.

It is possible to culture eye tissues so that successive generations of cells, which are susceptible to neoplastic change, can be studied. The use of a tissue culture system as well as epidemiologic data on squamous cell carcinoma of the eye of cattle are suggested for the study of radiation effects at the subcellular, cellular and whole animal levels.

Table III. Radioactive equilibrium between ^{210}Pb and [210]Po[b]

	Bovine choroid	
	[210]Pb [a]	[210]Po*
Chicago		
(Formalin preserved)	0·105 ± 0·126	1·886 ± 0·281
Minneapolis		
(Fresh)	0·358 ± 0·532	1·134 ± 0·184
	0·247 ± 0·154	0·349 ± 0·094
Boston		
(Fresh)	0·289 ± 0·204	0·144 ± 0·043
	0·247 ± 0·154	0·415 ± 0·183

[a] Expressed as pCi/g wet weight ± 2 SD.
[b] Analyses were done in cooperation with Northeastern Radiological Health Laboratory, U.S. Public Health Service.

Table IV.

		[210]Po [a]	[226]Ra [a]
MAN	Choroid and iris	0·027 ± 0·12	0·017 ± 0·005
	Retina	ND	0·006 ± 0·002
	Choroid and iris	0·272 ± 0·046	0·051 ± 0·015
	Retina	0·128 ± 0·045	0·025 ± 0·017
	Choroid and iris	0·015 ± 0·009	0·041 ± 0·011
	Retina	0·098 ± 0·017	0·034 ± 0·013
	Choroid and iris	0·024 ± 0·015	0·028 ± 0·006
	Retina	0	0·032 ± 0·026
MONKEY	Choroid and iris	0·731 ± 0·068	0·022 ± 0·022
	Choroid and iris	0·627 ± 0·049	0·104 ± 0·028
	Retina	0·879 ± 0·077	0
	Sclera	0·036 ± 0·008	0
DOG	Choroid and iris	0·740 ± 0·074	0·024 ± 0·008
	Choroid and iris	0·561 ± 0·042	0·065 ± 0·011
	Sclera	0·004 ± 0·004	0·005 ± 0·005
GOAT	Choroid	0·534 ± 0·050	0·018 ± 0·003
	Iris	0·616 ± 0·046	0·030 ± 0·006
	Retina	0·004 ± 0·002	0·001 ± 0·001
	Sclera	0·007 ± 0·006	0
FISH	Choroid and iris	0·359 ± 0·024	0·003 ± 0·001
(Haddock)	Choroid and iris	0·459 ± 0·035	0·013 ± 0·004
	Retina	0·274 ± 0·025	0·010 ± 0·004

[a] Expressed as pCi/g wet weight ± SD.
ND = not determined.

Acknowledgements.—This study has been supported by USPH Grant No. 5 PO1 ES-00002 and AEC Contract No. AT (30-1)-(3170). The Boston Eye Bank supplied human eyes for analysis.
Thanks are due to Dwyn Sherry and Clement Nelson who carried out the analyses.
Discussions with Dr. J. Shapiro have been most helpful.

REFERENCES

ANDERSON, D. E. (1963). Genetic aspects of cancer with special reference to cancer of the eye in the bovine. *Annals N.Y. Academy of Sciences* **108**, 948–62.

ANDERSON, D. E. and SKINNER, P. E. (1961). Studies on bovine ocular squamous carcinoma ("Cancer Eye"). XI. Effects of Sunlight. *J. Animal Science* **20**, 474–7.

BRANDLY, P. J. and MIGAKI, G. (1963). Types of tumors found by federal meat inspectors in an eight year survey. *Annals N.Y. Academy of Sciences* **108**, 872–9.

CHAPMAN, T. S. and HAMMONS, S., JR. (1963). Some observations concerning uranium content of ingesta and excreta of cattle. *Health Physics* **9**, 79–81.

COLE, L. J. and NOWELL, P. C. (1965). Radiation carcinogenesis. *Science* **150**, 1782–9.

DI FERRANTE, E. R. (1964). The natural concentration of ^{226}Ra in bovine bones and teeth. *Health Physics* **10**, 259–64.

DUDLEY, R. A. (1959). Natural and artificial radiation background of man. In *Low Level Irradiation,* Ed., A. M. Brues. AAAS Washington. 7–32.

ERLEKSOVA, E. V. (1960). *Raspredelenie nekotorykh radioaktivnykh elementov v organizme zhivotnykh (poloniya-210 radiotoriya 228, plutoniya 239, i strontsiya-90).* Atlas. Gosudarstvennoye izdatel'stvo meditsinskoy literatury Medgiz Moskva.

GARNER, R. J. (1963). Environmental contamination and grazing animals. *Health Physics* **9**, 597–605.

GRUNE, W. *et al.* (1960). *Natural Radioactivity in Ground Water Supplies in Maine and New Hampshire.* U.S. Public Health Service, Division of Radiological Health, Washington. Project No. A-473.

HILL, C. R. (1960). Lead 210 and polonium 210 in grass. *Nature* **187**, 211–12.

HILL, C. R. (1962). Identification of α- emitters in normal biological material. *Health Physics* **8**, 17–25.

HILL, C. R. and JAWOROWSKI, Z. S. (1961). Lead 210 in some human and animal tissues. *Nature* **190**, 353–4.

HOLTZMANN, R. B. (1963). *The Lead 210 Concentrations of some Biological Materials from Arctic Regions.* Radiological Physics Division Semi-annual Report. ANL 6769. pp. 59–65.

HOLTZMAN, R. B. (1963). Measurement of the natural contents of RaD (Pb 210) and RaF (Po 210) in human bone estimates of whole body burdens. *Health Physics* **9**, 385–400.

HOLTZMAN, R. B. (1964). Lead 210 and polonium 210 in potable waters in Illinois. In *The Natural Radiation Environment,* Ed. J. A. S. Adams and W. M. Lowder, Univ. of Chicago, Chicago. pp. 227–37.

HOLTZMAN, R. B. (1965). Lead 210 (RaD) in inhabitants of a Carribbean island. *Health Physics* **11**, 477–80.

HUNT, V. R., RADFORD, E. P., JR., and SEGALL, A. J. (1963). Comparison of concentrations of alpha-emitting elements in teeth and bones. *International Journal of Radiation Biology* **7**, 277–87.

HURSH, J. B. (1957). Natural occurrence of radium in man and in water and in food. *Brit. J. of Radiology,* Suppl. 7, 45–53.

LITTLE, J. B., RADFORD, E. P., JR., McCOMBS, H. L., HUNT, V. R., and NELSON, C. (1964). Polonium 210 in lungs and soft tissues of cigarette smokers. *Rad. Res.* **22**, 209 (Abstract).

LUCAS, H. F. and KRAUSE, D. G. (1960). Preliminary survey of Ra 226 and Ra 228 contents of drinking water. *Radiology* **74**, 114.

MAYNEORD, W. V. and HILL, C. R. (1959). Spectroscopic identification of alpha-emitting nuclides in biological material. *Nature* **184**, 667–9.

MONLUX, A. W., ANDERSON, W. A., and DAVIS, C. L. (1957). The diagnosis of squamous cell carcinoma of the eye ("Cancer Eye") in cattle. *Am. J. of Veterinary Research* **18**, 5–34.

PETROW, H. G., COVER, A., SCHIESSLE, W., and PARSONS, E. (1964). Radiochemical determination of Ra 228 and Th 228 in biological and mineral samples. *Analytical Chemistry* **36**, 1600–3.

PRINCE, J. H., DIESEM, C. D., EGLITIS, I. E., and RUSKELL, G. L. (1960). *Anatomy and Histology of the Eye and Orbit in Domestic Animals.* C. C. THOMAS, Springfield.

RADFORD, E. P., JR., HUNT, V. R., and SHERRY, D. (1963). Analysis of teeth and bones for alpha-emitting elements. *Rad. Res.* **19**, 298–315.

Recommendation of the International Commission of Radiological Protection (1955). *Brit. J. of Radiology,* Suppl. 6.

REHFELD, C. E., STOVER, B. J., TAYLOR, G. N., ATHERTON, D. R., and SCHNEEBELI, G. (1960). Eye changes in beagles following intravenous injection of Ra 226. *J. of Am. Veterinary Medicine Assn.* **136**, 562–4.

RUSSELL, W. O., WYNNE, E. S., and LOQUVAM, G. S. (1956). Studies on bovine ocular squamous carcinoma ("Cancer Eye"). *Cancer* **9**, 1–52.

STEINER, P. E., and BENGSTON, J. S. (1951). Research and economic aspects of tumors in food producing animals. *Cancer* **4**, 1113–24.

SYKES, J. A. L., DMOCHOWSKI, E. S., WYNNE, E. S., and RUSSELL, W. O. (1961). Bovine ocular squamous cell carcinoma. IV. Tissue culture studies of bovine ocular squamous-cell carcinoma and its benign precursor lesions. *J. Nat. Cancer Inst.* **26**, 445–87.

TRAUTMAN, A. and FIEBIGER, J. (1957). *The Fundamentals of the Histology of Domestic Animals.* Ithaca. N.Y.Comstock.

TSO, T. C., HALLDEN, N. A., and ALEXANDER, L. T. (1964). Radium 226 and polonium 210 in leaf tobacco and tobacco soil. *Science* **146**, 1043–5.

TRANSFER TO MILK OF INGESTED RADIOLEAD

R. E. STANLEY, A. A. MULLEN and E. W. BRETTHAUER

INTRODUCTION

THE RADIOLOGICAL health significance of environmental radionuclides is under continuing study at the Public Health Service's Southwestern Radiological Health Laboratory. Since dairy products, especially fresh milk, are one of the major links in the food chain by which radionuclides reach man, the dairy cow has been the animal of choice to evaluate the relative significance of the individual nuclides studied. The present study was undertaken to obtain the definitive biological data required to make a reliable assessment of the significance of a radiolead contaminated environment.

Radiolead is an activation product which may be released by the detonation of the nuclear explosives used in the Plowshare cratering program, a program to develop technology for the peaceful uses of nuclear explosives. Several radioisotopes of lead are produced by the neutron capture reaction with stable lead; however, the predominant isotope appearing in the environment is ^{203}Pb. Lead-203 has a substantially longer physical half-life than do the other gamma-emitting lead isotopes released, 2.2 days as compared to the next longest half-life of 3.6 hr. Lead-210, an alpha emitter having a long physical half-life, may be produced, but the reaction energies involved do not favor this production.

Although lead intoxication has been recognized as a disease entity for over 100 yr and has been studied extensively by numerous investigators, with the comprehensive work of KEHOE[1] and the review of JAWOROWSKI[2] as the more remarkable, data regarding the uptake and transfer by cows and other domestic ruminants are limited. Several investigators working with cows and sheep[3-5] report intestinal absorption ranging from essentially none to 1 or 2%. The human data[1] suggest that the amount of ingested lead absorbed may be as high as 8–10%. Other more recent data[6] from a one-cow study indicate that absorption may be less than 1% in the lactating cow.

In order to obtain more reliable biological data with which to assess the potential hazard imposed by Plowshare releases of radiolead, a study was conducted with four dairy cows which were given single oral doses of ^{203}Pb. In addition to the milk transfer data, this paper presents data on other compartment measurements, i.e., feces, urine and blood.

METHODS

The radioactive lead used in this study was prepared by Gulf General Atomics, San Diego, California. Stable lead, 61% abundant ^{204}Pb, was irradiated in a 25 MeV accelerator. After irradiation the lead was dissolved in dilute nitric acid and analyzed for radioactive content. Each ml of the resulting solution contained approximately 160 mg of lead and had a radioactive content of 731 μCi of ^{203}Pb, 5.05 μCi of ^{204}Pb, and 1.84 μCi of ^{202}Pb. Other than these three lead isotopes, no other radionuclides were detected in the solution. Since dosing of the cows did not occur until 9 hr later, the dosing solution was essentially all ²⁰³Pb (>99.5% pure).

The four Holstein cows used in this study were selected from the 20 cow milking herd of grade and purebred Holsteins maintained at the Nevada Test Site by the Public Health Service. The four cows, from 3 to 9 yr of age, were from 15 to 200 days into the current lactation period, and produced from 17 to 24 kg of milk daily. Throughout the study the cows were maintained on their regular ration, which was free access to water and alfalfa hay supplemented, at each milking, with a pelleted commercial dairy ration containing 16% protein.

For the major portion of the study (8 hr before to 126 hr after dosing) the cows were confined in metabolism stalls. These stalls facilitate total collection of feces and urine, permit access to either side for application of the milking machine, and are unrestrictive enough to allow the cows to lie down. Feces were collected in a grid-covered pan at the rear of the stall. An in-dwelling catheter inserted into the bladder of each cow and connected to a 20 l. bottle by plastic tubing was used for urine collection. Milking was accomplished with a milking machine and blood samples were taken periodically by jugular venipuncture. After the cows had been catheterized and allowed to become accustomed for 4 or 5 hr to the limited confinement of the metabolism stalls, samples of milk, feces, urine and blood were taken for background activity measurements.

Following the background collections, each cow was given 1.5 mCi of ²⁰³Pb dissolved in dilute nitric acid. The solution was contained in a ½ oz gelatin capsule which was placed inside a 1½ oz capsule for oral administration using a balling gun. Double encapsulation was used to minimize the possibility of capsule rupture during the dosing process. Total urine and fecal accumulations were collected every 6 hr for the duration of the cows' confinement in the stalls. A 400 ml. aliquot from each collection was placed in a plastic cottage cheese container and gamma counted. Blood samples and total milk accumulations were collected every 6 hr for the first 42 hr and every 12 hr thereafter for the duration of the study (197 hr after dosing for milk, 126 hr for all other excretion samples). A 400 ml. aliquot of each milk collection was also gamma counted. The blood samples, approximately 40 ml. collected at each milking, were gamma counted as whole blood, then centrifuged, and the serum portions counted separately. All counting was done using NaI (Tl) crystals connected to single-channel analyzers set on the 0.279 MeV peak of ²⁰³Pb. Samples were counted for up to 40 min and sample collection was stopped when the counting error exceeded 30%.

RESULTS

The ²⁰³Pb concentrations in milk are shown in Fig. 1, plotted as a function of time and decay corrected both to time of administration and to time of collection. The data were expressed as per cent of the administered dose and averaged for the four cows used in the study. The biological and effective half-lives were determined by least squares fit of the data. The peak activity concentration appeared in the milk 30 hr after the administration of the ²⁰³Pb and represented 0.0003% of the administered dose per liter. The biological half-life of lead as measured in milk was 70.4 hr. Correspondingly, the effective half-life in this compartment for ²⁰³Pb was 29.9 hr,

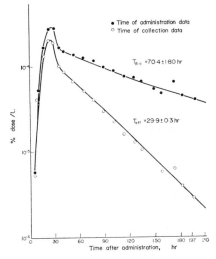

FIG. 1. Decay corrected ²⁰³Pb concentrations in milk, average data for four cows.

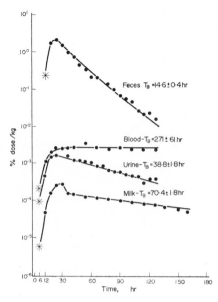

FIG. 2. ²⁰³Pb concentrations in feces, urine, blood, and milk decay corrected to time of administration.

with peak activity at time of collection of 0.0002 % of the dose per liter of milk.

Figure 2 shows the distribution of the lead among the feces, blood, urine and milk. Peak concentrations, corrected to the time of administration, were observed at 24 hr after dosing for the feces and urine, 30 hr for the milk, and 54 hr for the blood. Expressed as percent of dose, the respective peak concentrations for feces, urine, milk and blood were 2.12, 0.0017, 0.0003 and 0.0027 %. Also note in this figure, that activity was detected at 6 hr in all compartments except feces. Activity first appeared in the feces sometime during the interval between the 6 and 12 hr collections.

Table 1 presents the total excretion and secretion percentages as a function of time. The peak outputs in the feces and urine occurred at 18 hr, 6 hr earlier than the concentration peaks in these two compartments. The peak total activity secreted in milk was observed at 30 hr,

the same time as was recorded for the peak concentration. More than 50 % of the administered dose was excreted during the first 30 hr after dosing and at 42 hr, greater than 75 % had been excreted. For the total time that the cows were confined in the metabolism stalls, 126 hr or approximately 5 days, 93 % of the administered ²⁰³Pb had been recovered. Of the amount recovered during this period, more than 99 % was recovered in the feces. Approximately 6.5 times as much activity was excreted in the urine as was secreted in the milk. However, the combined urine and milk pathways accounted for less than 1 % of the recovered nuclide.

At the first sampling period, 6 hr after dosing, the blood activity concentration was 3.35 nCi per l. or approximately 0.0002 % of the administered dose. The peak concentration of 47 nCi was observed at 54 hr and represented 0.003 % of the dose. The levels changed only slightly for the remainder of the study with 30 nCi per liter measured at 178 hr after dosing. Most of the activity was associated with the formed elements, probably the erythrocytes. Measurable activity was found in the serum at only six sampling times beginning at the 12 hr collection and disappearing after the 42 hr collection.

The peak serum concentration appeared at 24 hr; however, the 1.9 nCi per l. was less than 5 % of the activity measured in the whole blood at this collection. Table 2 shows the blood to serum relationship at all samplings where activity was detected in the serum.

DISCUSSION

The results of this study tend to support the findings of other investigators[3–5] that lead is sparingly absorbed in the gastro-intestinal tract. Although the lead nitrate used in this study is one of the more soluble salts of inorganic lead, this property apparently exerts little influence on gut absorption. GARNER[4] saw little difference between the absorption of lead acetate, a soluble salt, and the carbonate form which is relatively insoluble. KEHOE's[1] experience was much the same in that he detected little difference between ingested soluble and insoluble lead. This is probably due to the formation of relatively insoluble complexes with proteins

116

Table 1. Total ^{203}Pb output (urine, milk and feces) as % administered dose recovered*

Elapsed time (hr)	(%) in feces	(%) in urine	(%) in milk	Total (%) out	Cumul. (%) out
0					
6	0.0	0.0008	0.00003	0.0008	
12	2.48	0.0051	0.00039	2.49	2.49
18	19.5	0.0122	0.00078	19.51	22.0
24	18.8	0.0105	0.00134	18.81	40.81
30	18.4	0.0109	0.00229	18.41	59.22
36	10.2	0.0088	0.00106	10.21	69.43
42	7.34	0.0083	0.00103	7.35	76.78
48	4.12	0.0072		4.13	80.91
54	3.42	0.0075	0.00178	3.43	84.34
60	2.06	0.0063		2.07	86.41
66	1.52	0.0060	0.00113	1.53	87.94
72	1.13	0.0044		1.13	89.07
78	1.22	0.0052	0.00151	1.23	90.3
84	0.85	0.0039		0.854	91.15
90	0.56	0.0061	0.00097	0.567	91.72
96	0.31	0.0042		0.314	92.03
102	0.42	0.0041	0.00106	0.425	92.46
108	0.23	0.0032		0.233	92.69
114	0.19	0.0031	0.00079	0.194	92.88
120	0.18	0.0035		0.184	93.07
126	0.12	0.0030	0.00073	0.124	93.19
Totals	93.05	0.124	0.0149	93.19	

* The data are average values for the four cows and are decay corrected to the time of administration.

Table 2. Average activity concentrations in blood and serum

Time after dosing	Whole blood (nCi/l)	Serum (nCi/l)
6 hrs	3.35	Not detected
12	16.8	0.22
18	29.4	0.33
24	40.0	1.91
30	40.7	0.26
36	41.4	0.25
42	42.8	0.24
54	47.0	Not detected
178 (7 days)	30.4	Not detected

and other compounds within the intestinal tract. Therefore, no matter what form ingested the forms presented for absorption are the "insoluble" complexes.

The peak activity concentrations in urine and milk, the two compartments whose activity results from the absorbable fraction of the nuclide, occurred at 24–30 hr after dosing and are related to the peak in the serum at 24 hr. Apparently, the radioactivity in the serum is the portion of the circulating activity which is readily exchangeable with the two excretory compartments. The later peak in the whole blood at 54 hr appeared to have little influence on the diminishing transfer rate to milk and urine. The results of this study showed that more than 95% of the blood activity was associated with the formed elements, probably incorporated in the erythrocytes, and are similar to Kehoe's[1] findings. Apparently, the erythrocytic bound or incorporated activity is not readily exchangeable.

Although the fraction deposited in the bone was not determined in this study, the results can be generally applied to evaluate the significance of other types of radiolead releases in which ^{210}Pb might be the predominant isotope for radiological health consideration. Based on the ratio of absorbed lead to that secreted in the milk, the increased milk fraction resulting from

117

the mobilization of the deposited ^{210}Pb would be small. The potential increased significance of ^{210}Pb is further reduced when considering the large fraction of circulating lead which was incorporated in the red cells and apparently not readily transferable. Presumably the incorporated lead would remain with the erythrocytes until their destruction occurs. After erythrocytic destruction a certain fraction of the sequestered lead would be removed by the liver and excreted in the bile to the feces. Hence, any additional significance from ^{210}Pb by the milk pathway to man would be limited.

Based on the results of this study, radiolead released by Plowshare explosives does not appear to be a significant radionuclide for radiological health consideration. Ingested lead is only sparingly absorbed by the dairy cow. The preferred excretory pathway for the cow of the circulating transferable portion is the urine. One-sixth of the amount excreted in the urine is secreted in the milk and the milk portion represents only 0.02 per cent of the total ingested lead. The significance is further minimized when considering the conditions of generation and the relative short half-life of the principal lead isotope produced.

REFERENCES

1. R. A. KEHOE, Industrial lead poisoning, *Industrial hygiene and Toxicology*, 2nd Edition, pp. 941–985. Wiley Interscience, New York (1965).
2. Z. JAWOROWSKI, Radioactive lead in the environment and in the human body. *G.E.C. atom. Energy Rev.* Vol. VII, No. 1. (1969).
3. S. P. MARSHALL, F. W. HAYWARD and W. R. MEAGHER, Effects of feeding arsenic and lead upon their secretion in milk. *J. Dairy Sci.* **46,** 580 (1963).
4. R. J. GARNER, *Veterinary Toxicology*, 2nd Edition, pp. 94–101. Williams and Wilkens, Baltimore (1963).
5. K. L. BAXTER, Lead as a nutritional hazard to farm livestock. II. The absorption and excretion of lead by sheep and rabbits. *J. comp. Path. Ther.* **60,** 140 (1950).
6. G. POTTER, Biological availability of ^{203}Pb and ^{204}Tl in the dairy cow and calf. Lawrence Radiation Lab. Memo. Rep., 14 August (1969).

The Fate and Implications of ²⁰³Pb Ingestion in a Dairy Cow and a Calf

G. D. POTTER
D. R. McINTYRE
G. M. VATTUONE

Introduction

MOST of the current interest in lead metabolism is related to its toxic properties and to lead poisoning. There is a vast amount of literature on lead toxicity and lead metabolism; excellent reviews are presented in most major pharmacology texts.[1–3] Lead is widely distributed in nature and readily forms organic compounds with many plants. Lead poisoning is probably the most common form of metallic poisoning in livestock throughout the world.[3]

Lead is not absorbed through the intact skin but most of its compounds are absorbable from mucous membranes and exposed tissues.[1] The principal routes of entry are the digestive and respiratory systems. Lead must be in solution before it can be absorbed, but even the most "insoluble" lead salts and metallic lead, if finely divided, are somewhat soluble in the digestive juices and tissues; the "soluble" salts are to a great extent precipitated. The greater part of ingested lead, soluble as well as "insoluble," is unabsorbed. Lead poisoning often develops more rapidly with inhalation than by other methods since inhaled lead is more finely divided.[2] Inorganic compounds of lead (except the silicate) are dissolved in gastric juice and are readily converted to the chloride. In the large intestine a portion of the unabsorbed lead is converted into the sulfide.[2] Thus most forms of inorganic lead which are ingested would be expected to behave in a similar manner. Tetraethyl lead is absorbed from the lungs, skin, and digestive tract. Its early distribution differs from that of the water-soluble compounds, but it is decomposed by tissues and is then distributed as water-soluble lead and acts as such.[2]

Lead is concentrated in bone, liver, kidney and red blood cells.[1] After it is orally administered, it is excreted primarily in the feces, in the form of unabsorbed lead plus that excreted in the bile and through the intestinal mucosa.[3] It is also eliminated in urine, but apparently there is an upper limit for this route. However, when blood levels are high, the rate of excretion is increased out of proportion to the concentration, possibly as a result of reduced degree of binding to erythrocytes or of saturating of binding sites.[1] The concentrations of lead in milk appear to be proportional to those in the blood cells.[3]

These well-known features of lead metabolism are pertinent to the uptake, distribution, and removal of radioactive lead in the mammalian system. Assuming high-energy neutrons incident on lead, the nuclear reactions involved in the production of ^{210}Pb are multiple n, λ reactions with stable lead (^{206}Pb through ^{208}Pb), while ^{203}Pb could be produced from multiple n, 2n reactions with ^{204}Pb through ^{208}Pb. Similar reactions of this type have been documented elsewhere.[4] The experiments described here were done to study the internal transport and biological availability of radioactive lead that could be produced and released in certain types of nuclear cratering events, especially ^{203}Pb (52 hr) and ^{210}Pb (22 hr). The latter probably is more important biologically because of its long half-life and radioactive daughters, while the former decays to stable ^{203}Tl.

Methods

The methods used here are essentially those described previously.[5] A lactating Holstein dairy cow (weight 749 kg) from the LRL dairy herd was used for the metabolic experiment and a 68.3-kg calf for the tissue distribution study. Carrier-free radioactive lead (^{203}Pb) as $Pb(NO_3)_2$ was absorbed into anhydrous glucose in gelatine veterinarian capsules and administered with a balling gun. The cow was fed 5.2 mCi and the calf 3.0 mCi of the ^{203}Pb.

The cow was maintained in a metabolic stall with free access to alfalfa hay and water for the duration of the experiment (144 hr) plus an additional supplement of 3 kg of commercial dairy mix at each milking. Urine was collected by means of an internal catheter; feces were collected in a stainless steel collection pan; milking was done with Surge equipment. In each case, samples were pooled for each 24-hr period. The pooled feces were blended in a large dough mixer to reduce inhomogeneities. For counting, 200-g samples of milk, urine and feces were placed in aluminum tuna cans. All samples had 4–5 ml of 40% formalin added as a preservative. A 2% solution of agar was

120

Table 1. *Recovery of orally administered ^{203}Pb administered as $Pb(NO_3)_2$ (as percentage of administered dose) to a lactating dairy cow*

Collection time (hr)	Feces (%)	Feces (%)/kg	Urine (%)	Urine (%)/kg	Milk (%)	Milk (%)/kg	Plasma (%)/kg	RBC (%)/kg
24	42.1	0.958	0.022	0.00119	0.00180	0.00015	0.00015	0.00695
48	42.6	1.17	0.047	0.00225	0.00414	0.00037	0.00008	0.00948
72	7.36	0.207	0.036	0.00178	0.00385	0.00031	0.00008	0.01010
96	1.75	0.055	0.025	0.00173	0.00300	0.00025	0.00009	0.00918
120	0.552	0.023	0.022	0.00145	0.00243	0.00021	0.00005	0.00791
144	0.214	0.0061	0.021	0.00128	0.00173	0.00019	0.00002	0.00652
Total	94.576		0.173		0.0170			
Total recovered	94.768							

added as a preservative. A 2% solution of agar was added as needed to keep particulate matter distributed in the cans to maintain standard counting geometry. The cans were sealed with a hand sealer. Blood samples (500 ml) were withdrawn at 24-hr intervals, following morning milking, heparinized, and centrifuged in a refrigerated centrifuge. Plasma was separated from the cells and canned for counting. The cells were then combined and recentrifuged; the remaining plasma was withdrawn and discarded, and the cells were canned for counting.

All samples were counted between a pair of 4 ×4 in. NaI(Tl) crystals with a single-channel analyzer with a window set to detect the photon resulting from K-electron capture of thallium at about 72 keV. Integrated counts were recorded for each sample. The data obtained were processed by computer, using a code specially devised for this purpose.

The calf had free access to chopped alfalfa hay and water with an additional ration of 1 kg of calf starter each day. It was anesthetized 42.5 hr after administration of the [203]Pb and exsanguinated after collection of a large heparinized blood sample. Representative organs and tissues were removed and weighed, and 200-g samples were canned. Tissues that weighed less than 200 g were minced and 2% agar was added to make up 200 g. Formalin was also added to these samples. The cans were sealed and counted as described above. The data were processed by computer with a code similar to that used for analysis of the metabolic by-products. All samples were corrected for physical decay to the time of administration.

Results

Figure 1 and Table 1 give the excretion and blood data from the cow. Figure 1 shows the recovery of [203]Pb as a percentage of the administered dose versus time for milk, urine, feces, plasma and blood cells. Figure 2 shows the calculated body burden of [203]Pb in the cow as a function of time.

Table 2 shows the distribution of [203]Pb in calf tissues as tissue-to-plasma (T/P) ratios, percentages of the administered dose per kg of tissue, and total recoveries as percentages of administered dose.

Discussion

The data in Table 1 show a total recovery of 94.768% of the [203]Pb in the feces, urine and milk of the cow by 144 hr. Approximately 85% was recovered in the feces in the first 48 hr. The total secretion in urine during 144 hr was 0.173%, while the total secretion in milk was 0.190. These results appear to confirm the literature on the slow, incomplete absorp-

122

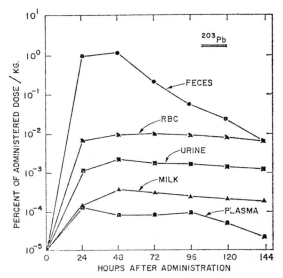

Fig. 1. The concentrations of ^{203}Pb in milk, urine, feces, plasma and red blood cells following oral administration to a lactating cow.

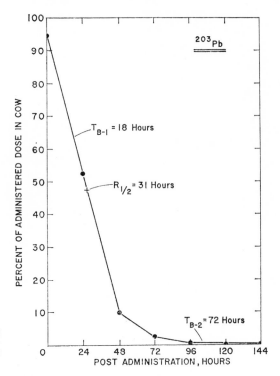

FIG. 2. The whole-body burden of ^{203}Pb administered orally to a lactating cow. Points were calculated by subtracting from the administered dose the total recovery (94.8%) of ^{203}Pb in milk, urine and feces.

$R_{1/2}$ = half-retention time,
T_{B-1} = biological half-time for fast component,
T_{B-2} = biological half-time of slow component.

tion of lead from the digestive tract.[1-3] However, since absorbed lead is excreted even more slowly, a low-level, continuous administration is associated with gradual accumulation so that eventually clinical poisoning becomes apparent. Since lead, like other heavy metals, has an affinity for sulfur, it combines with sulfhydryl groups. It is usually considered to exert its effects through sulfhydryl inhibition, but the fact that it is deposited in bone salts demonstrates that it has other affinities *in vivo* and may interact also with carboxyl, phosphoryl, and other groups.[1]

Figure 1 shows the rapid elimination of ^{203}Pb in the feces and its slow elimination in blood cells, plasma, urine and milk. It is also of interest that the level in blood cells is about two orders of magnitude higher than that in plasma, but less than an order of magnitude higher than in urine.

Figure 2 represents the whole-body burden of ^{203}Pb in the cow, calculated by subtracting from the administered dose the sum of the activities of the excretory products at each 24-hr point. The lead-retention curve has two distinct components, an early fast component with a biological half-time of 18 hr primarily reflecting fecal elimination and a slow component with a half-time of about 72 hr reflecting elimination of absorbed lead via urine and milk as well as a proportionately large amount of residual radioactivity in feces (Fig. 1 and Table 1). The half-residence time in the cow was 31 hr.

The tissue distribution of the absorbed lead in the calf is shown in Table 2. In blood the largest fraction is associated with the erythrocytes; the T/P ratio is 122. The total recovery values show that the erythrocytes represent the largest pool of lead next to liver and bone (T/P ratios 263 and 44.5, respectively). Kidney also has a high T/P ratio (235), but the total amount is less because of the smaller mass of tissue.[1] The tissue data from the calf confirm the known pattern of distribution of inorganic lead in soft tissues, with the highest concentrations in liver and kidneys. It is well known that over a period of time, it is redistributed and deposited principally in bone and in teeth.

The production and release of radiolead to the environment from certain nuclear reactions leads to consideration of possible counter-measures for its removal. Its behaviour resembles that of another divalent cation, calcium, which is deposited as insoluble tertiary lead phosphate in bone.[6]

Factors that affect calcium metabolism similarly affect that of lead,[1] i.e., high phosphate intake favors skeletal storage and reduces the levels in soft tissue. Conversely, low phosphate intake mobilizes lead in bone and increases its concentration in soft tissues. Calcium competes with lead for available phosphate. Such other factors as Vitamin D, parathyroid hormone, dihydrotachysterol, acidosis, iodides and bicarbonate all affect the deposition or mobilization of lead in bone. Since lead deposited in bone salts does not contribute to lead toxicity, the treatment of acute intoxication would involve procedures that favor skeletal storage of lead. At later stages lead is mobilized from the bones to urine by manipulating the calcium phosphate intake and administration of acidifying salts or other agents to promote its removal. However, these procedures must be used cautiously to prevent the recurrence of the acute toxicity syndrome.[1] Ethylenediaminetetraacetate (EDTA) has

125

Table 2. Distribution of [203]Pb in tissues of a calf 42 hr after oral administration of $Pb(NO_3)_2$

Tissue	T/P ratio	Concentration %/kg‡	Recovery (% per organ)‡
Plasma	1.000	0.005	0.001
Liver	263.	0.345	0.394
Kidney	235.	0.308	0.105
Erythrocytes	122.	0.161	0.236*
Bone (mixed)	44.5	0.058	0.374*
Compact bone	23.9	0.031	—
Spleen	16.9	0.022	0.004
Lung	13.7	0.018	0.013
Marrow	13.1	0.017	—
Bile	11.4	0.015	—
Thyroid	9.69	0.013	—
Thymus	9.34	0.012	0.001
Salivary	6.43	0.008	0.001
Testes	5.13	0.007	—
Cartilage	4.06	0.005	—
Fat	3.07	0.004	—
Heart	2.65	0.003	0.001
Brain	1.54	0.002	0.001
Muscle	0.799	0.001	0.001*
Total recovered			1.132†

* Total weights estimated as percentage of total body weight.

† Excluding integument, gastrointestinal tract and contents, and organs for which no values are given (could not be estimated or values were too low for inclusion in table).

‡ Percentages are percentage of administered dose.

been shown to be a most effective chelating agent for treatment of lead poisoning, but its administration must be carefully controlled since it is not highly selective for lead, and its avidity for calcium (and other divalent cations) could result in a fatal hypocalcemia. To minimize this problem EDTA is administered as the calcium chelate (Ca EDTA). This treatment reduces the soft tissue burden but does not affect lead deposited in bone.[3] These same therapeutic procedures would be indicated in the treatment of individuals having large body burdens of radioactive lead. Dimercaprol (BAL) is of little value in the treatment of lead poisoning in animals; there is some evidence that it may increase the renal toxicity of lead.

Acknowledgement—This work was performed under the auspices of the U.S.A.E.C. Reference to a company or product name does not imply approval or recommendation of the product by the U.S.A.E.C. or the University of California over others that may be suitable.

References

1. L. S. GOODMAN and A. GILMAN, *The Pharmacological bases of Therapeutics*, 3rd edition. Macmillan, New York (1965).
2. T. SOLLMAN, *A Manual of Pharmacology and its applications to Therapeutics and Toxicology*. W. B. Saunders and Co. (1957).
3. L. M. JONES, *Veterinary Pharmacology and Toxicology*, 3rd edition. Iowa State University Press, Ames, Iowa (1965).
4. H. TEWES, Radioactivity source terms for underground engineering application. Proc. Symp. on Public Health Aspects of Peaceful Uses of Nuclear Explosives. U.S. Dep. of Hlth, Education and Welfare, SWRHL-82, pp. 207–222 (1969).
5. G. D. POTTER, J. M. VATTUONE and D. R. McINTYRE, The metabolism of ^{204}Tl administered as TlNO$_3$ in the dairy cow and calf. Lawrence Radiation Lab., Livermore, Rep. UCRL-72350 (1970).
6. R. F. GUYMER, The metabolism of lead in man in health and disease, The Harben Lectures 1960, *Jl. R. Inst. publ. Hlth.* **24,** 101 (1961).

Reduction of Lead Absorption from the Intestine in Newborn Rats

K. Kostial, I. Šimonović, and M. Pišonić

We have recently shown that the absorption of lead, like the absorption of other cations, is very high in newborn rats (Kostial et al., 1971). This might be an important factor in human babies and small children who are generally believed to be more exposed to oral lead poisoning and who are also supposed to be more sensitive to lead poisoning than adults (Barltrop, 1969).

The purpose of our work was to evaluate whether this high absorption of lead from the intestine can be reduced by various additives to the milk. First of all we wanted to estimate the effect of calcium and phosphate additives to the milk. Earlier investigations have indicated that calcium and phosphorus in the diet influence deposition of lead in soft tissue and bone (Sobel et al., 1940). Recently Six and Goyer (1970) have shown that the lowering of calcium in the diet increases the toxicity of lead in rats. This might not apply to very young animals with a much higher lead absorption from the intestine. The addition of considerable amounts of calcium and phosphate to the milk had no effect on the percentage calcium or strontium absorption from the intestine in newborn rats (Kostial et al., 1969).

The effect of alginates on the absorption of lead from the gut was estimated in humans and rats (Harrison et al., 1969; Carr et al., 1969). Although these results show no or only a small effect of alginates on lead absorption in humans and rats on normal diet, there is some indication that alginates might cause a decrease in lead absorption in rats fed a milk diet (Carr et al., 1969).

Since none of these experiments has been performed in very young animals, our present study has been entirely carried out on newborn rats. A method similar to that in our previous study on calcium and strontium absorption in newborn rats was used (Kostial et al., 1967). Our results indicate that calcium, phosphate, and alginate additives to the milk cause a considerable reduction in the body burden of lead in newborn rats.

MATERIALS AND METHODS

The experiment was performed on 5–7-day-old baby rats which were artifically fed over a period of 8 hours with cow's milk and with milk to which calcium, phosphate, and alginate were added. The animals were divided into three groups. In the first group the rats were fed on cow's milk with an average content of 140 mg Ca and 95 mg P/100 ml. In the second group the rats received cow's milk to which calcium chloride and potassium dehydrogen phosphate were added to reach the level of rat's milk with an average content of 400 mg Ca and 230 mg P/100 ml (Widdowson and Dickerson, 1964). The third group received the equivalent of rat's milk and an addition of 2 g of sodium alginate O.G.1. (Humphreys, 1967) per 100 ml.

Carrier-free lead-203 (supplied as a chloride by the Gustaf Werner Institute, University of Uppsala, Sweden) was added in tracer amounts to the milk in all groups. Each animal received, over the 8-hour artificial feeding period, on the average, 0.45 ml of milk in 17 drops containing about 2 μCi of lead-203.

In some experiments carrier-free calcium-47 (supplied as a chloride from the Radiochemical Center, Amersham, England) was also added to the milk in amounts of 1 μCi per animal.

Immediately after the artificial feeding period the baby rats were returned to their mothers where they stayed until sacrifice 90 hours after the beginning of the experiment. The lead-203 and calcium-47 content in the whole body was determined before and after removal of the intestinal tract in a two scintillation counter assembly connected to a single channel analyzer. The results were expressed as percentages of the oral dose retained in the body.

The lead-203 retention was also determined in the kidney and liver in a well-type scintillation counter after estimating the wet weight of these organs. The activity of calcium-47 was too low to be estimated. The results were expressed as percentage of the dose retained in the kidneys or liver per 1 gram of wet weight of these organs.

RESULTS

The retention of lead-203 and calcium-47 in the body before and after removal of the intestinal tract is presented in Table 1. All retention values for lead-203 were lower after removal of the intestinal tract. The retention values for calcium-47 in the body were, however, practically the same before and after removal of the intestinal tract.

The highest retention values were observed in the group of animals fed on cow's milk with the lower calcium and phosphate content (Tables 1 and 2). The retention of lead-203 in the body, kidney, and liver was about 1.4 times lower in animals with calcium and phosphate milk additives and approximately 2.5 times lower in animals with calcium, phosphate, and alginate additives.

DISCUSSION

The high retention values in the body of newborn animals after ingestion of lead-203 are entirely in agreement with our previous results (Kostial et al., 1971) indicating that our present estimates of the percentage lead absorption from the intestine might be much too low for this age group.

TABLE 1
THE INFLUENCE OF CALCIUM, PHOSPHORUS, AND ALGINATE MILK ADDITIVES ON
RETENTION OF RADIOACTIVE LEAD AND CALCIUM IN THE BODY OF
5-7-DAY-OLD ARTIFICIALLY FED RATS

Milk (mg/100 ml)			% Ingested dose in the body			
			With intestinal tract		Without intestinal tract	
Ca	P	Alginate	^{203}Pb	^{47}Ca	^{203}Pb	^{47}Ca
140	95	—	82.35 ± 1.71 (54)[a]	78.53 ± 1.39 (12)	73.41 ± 1.92	77.82 ± 1.55
400	230	—	61.70 ± 1.05 (53)	78.35 ± 1.97 (12)	54.50 ± 1.03	75.48 ± 1.68
400	230	2000	34.97 ± 2.31 (54)	61.93 ± 2.05 (24)	24.68 ± 1.61	64.65 ± 2.45

[a] Figures in parentheses indicate the number of animals in a group. The results are expressed as arithmetic means ± standard error of the means.

We can assume that the retention values obtained before the removal of the intestinal tract are a better indication of the percentage absorption, since the values obtained in the intestinal tract at the time of sacrifice are most probably partly due to the endogenous fecal secretion (which is the main route of lead excretion from the body) and partly to the radioactive lead content in the intestinal wall. It is not likely that any unabsorbed fraction of lead was still present in the intestine at the time of sacrifice, since calcium-47 retention values were practically the same before and after removal of the intestinal tract, indicating that the unabsorbed fraction had already been removed from the body by fecal excretion.

From this experiment we cannot conclude whether an increased calcium or phosphate content of the milk causes a reduction in lead absorption from the intestinal tract. Therefore any speculations as to the mechanism of this action would not be justified. In one case the effect might be due to a competitive action of calcium ions in the transfer of lead through the intestinal wall (Six and Goyer, 1970) and in the other case the formation of insoluble lead phosphate might be an explanation. It is interesting to notice that an increase of calcium and phosphates in the milk caused no changes in the percentage calcium absorption from the intestine indicating a greatly increased total calcium absorption as observed in our earlier experiments (Kostial *et al.*, 1967; Kostial *et al* 1969).

TABLE 2
THE INFLUENCE OF CALCIUM, PHOSPHORUS, AND ALGINATE MILK ADDITIVES ON THE
RETENTION OF RADIOACTIVE LEAD IN THE LIVER AND KIDNEY OF 5-7-DAY OLD
ARTIFICIALLY FED RATS

Milk (mg/100 ml)			No. of animals	Lead-203 percentage ingested dose/1 g wet tissue	
Ca	P	Alginate		Liver	Kidney
140	95	—	54	5.39 ± 0.23	2.98 ± 0.08
400	230	—	53	3.64 ± 0.17	2.13 ± 0.11
400	230	2000	54	2.15 ± 0.15	1.16 ± 0.09

The fact that alginates cause a selective reduction of lead absorption could be explained by the stronger binding of lead to alginates as shown by the inotropic series quoted by Haug (1960). However, why this effect of alginates was not observed in animals or humans on normal diet (Harrison et al., 1969; Carr et al., 1969) remains to be explained.

It is also interesting to note that the retention in the kidneys expressed as percentages of the dose per gram of tissue is about 2 times lower than the retention in the liver, while adult animals retain about 6–10 times more lead in the kidney than in the liver at similar time intervals (Castellino and Aloj, 1964). This might indicate a different distribution of lead in relation to age, but more data at different time intervals are necessary to prove this hypothesis.

The finding that the very high lead absorption from the intestine in the very young could be decreased by additives which have up to now proved to be harmless in rats and humans (Harrison, 1967) might be interesting since there is already some evidence that appreciable body burdens of lead may be acquired by children (Barltrop, 1969).

REFERENCES

BARLTROP, D. (1969). Environmental lead and its paediatric significance. *Postgrad. Med. J.* **45**, 129–134.

CARR, T. E. F., NOLAN, J., AND DURAKOVIĆ, A. (1969). Effect of alginate on the absorption and excretion of ^{203}Pb in rats fed milk and normal diets. *Nature London* **224**, 1115.

CASTELLINO, N., AND ALOJ, S. (1964). Kinetics of the distribution and excretion of lead in the rat. *Brit. J. Ind. Med.* **21**, 308–314.

HARRISON, G. E. (1967). Absorption of strontium in rats on alginate supplemented diet. *In* "Diagnosis and Treatment of Deposited Radionuclides," (H. A. Kornberg and W. D. Norwood, eds.), pp. 333–339. Excerpta Medica Foundation, Amsterdam.

HARRISON, G. E., CARR, T. E. F., SUTTON, A., AND HUMPHREYS, E. R. (1969). Effect of alginate on the absorption of lead in man *Nature London* **224**, 1115–1116.

HAUG, R. (1960). Report No. 30. Composition and properties of alginates, p. 47. Norwegian Institute of Seaweed Research, Trondheim.

HUMPHREYS, E. R. (1967). Preparation of an oligoguluronide from sodium alginate. *Carbohyd. Res.* **4**, 507–509.

KOSTIAL, K., DURAKOVIĆ, A., ŠIMONOVIĆ, I., AND JUVANČIĆ, V. (1969). The effect of some dietary additives on calcium and strontium absorption in suckling and lactating rats. *Int. J. Radiat. Biol.* **15**, 563–570.

KOSTIAL, K., ŠIMONOVIĆ, I., AND PIŠONIĆ, M. (1967). Effect of calcium and phosphate on gastrointestinal absorption of strontium and calcium in newborn rats. *Nature London* **215**, 1181–1182.

KOSTIAL, K., ŠIMONOVIĆ, I., AND PIŠONIĆ, M. (1971). Lead absorption from the intestine in newborn rats. Communication at the III Yugoslav Congress of Industrial Medicine, Lijubljana.

SIX, K. M., AND GOYER, R. A. (1970). Experimental enhancement of lead toxicity by low dietary calcium. *J. Lab Clin. Med.* **76**, 933–940.

SOBEL, A. E., YUSKA, H., PETERS, D..D., AND KRAMER, B. (1940). The biochemical behaviour of lead. 1. Influence of calcium, phosphorus and vitamin D on lead in blood and bone. *J. Biol. Chem.* **132**, 239–265.

WIDDOWSON, E. M., AND DICKERSON, J. W. T. (1964). Chemical composition of the body. *In* "Mineral Metabolism" (C. L. Comar and F. Bronner, eds.), Vol. 2A, pp. 2–207. Academic Press, New York.

Cellular Effects Of Lead
And Lead Metabolites

Ion Transport by Heart Mitochondria

XXIII. The Effects of Lead on Mitochondrial Reactions

K. M. SCOTT, K. M. HWANG, M. JURKOWITZ, AND G. P. BRIERLEY

Alterations in the structure and function of mitochondria in various tissues have been observed after lead poisoning *in vivo*, and the mitochondrion appears to be one of the potential sites for the toxic effects of lead (1–7). Our continued interest in the effects of heavy-metal ions on isolated beef heart mitochondria has led us to investigate the effects of lead on these organelles as a possible model for the interaction of this cation with biological membranes. In the present report we wish to summarize a number of the effects of lead on mitochondrial permeability, on ion transport reactions, and on respiration.

METHODS

Beef heart mitochondria were prepared using Nagarse and EGTA[1] as previously described (8).

[1] The abbreviations used are as follows: CMB, p-chloromercuribenzoate; CMS, p-chloromercuri-

Respiration, pH, and changes in absorbancy at 546 mμ (swelling and contraction) were monitored simultaneously in the Eppendorf photometer modified as previously described (9, 10). In a number of experiments the swelling was also shown by the increase in water content of sedimented mitochondrial pellets (11). The binding of Pb^{2+} to the mitochondrion was determined by atomic absorption spectroscopy of supernatant fluids after removal of mitochondria by either centrifugation or filtration through Millipore filters.

Changes in Pb^{2+} concentration were also followed by the dual-wavelength technique using an Aminco–Chance instrument and the multiple-parameter cell as published (12). Absorbance changes of the Pb^{2+}-sensitive indicator murexide were monitored at 540 mμ using 510 mμ as a reference wavelength as described by Mela (13) for

phenyl sulfonate; CCP, *m*-chlorocarbonylcyanidephenylhydrazone; TMPD, N,N,N',N'-tetramethylphenylenediamine; EGTA, ethyleneglycol bis (aminoethyl) tetraacetic acid.

Ca²⁺ measurements. Pb²⁺ uptake as measured in this way agreed well with the corresponding value obtained by atomic absorption. The interaction of Ca²⁺ with the dye is sufficiently less sensitive that Ca²⁺ does not interfere with the Pb²⁺ estimation. Changes in the absorbance of bromthymol blue (14, 15) as an indication of membrane pH changes were recorded with 618 mμ as the measuring and 700 mμ as the reference wavelength.

Succinic dehydrogenase was determined in the presence of antimycin using phenazine methosulfate as electron acceptor, essentially as described by King (16). Submitochondrial particles were prepared by sonication in the absence of added chelators or other additions as described by Jacobus and Brierley (17).

The release of K⁺ from mitochondria was followed at 25° in a stirred glass chamber fitted with a Lucite plug which was machined to hold a Sargent S-30070 micro-combination pH electrode, a Clark oxygen electrode (YSI 5331), and a Beckman 39047 cation-sensitive electrode. The pH and cation-sensitive electrodes were plugged to a common reference and responded only to additions of H⁺ or K⁺, respectively, without cross interaction. The composition of the various suspending media and other experimental conditions are given with the individual experiments reported.

RESULTS

Passive binding of lead by isolated heart mitochondria. The anionic composition of the suspending medium strongly affects the amount of lead which is bound by mitochondria in the absence of metabolic energy. Determination of lead binding by either the atomic-absorption or the murexide procedures shows that most of the added lead is bound in a medium of KCl or KNO₃ in the range from 0 to 40 μM lead (Fig. 1). As more lead is added, the binding capacity becomes saturated at a value near 140 nmoles of lead per milligram of protein. Scatchard plots of lead-binding data under these conditions are biphasic and closely resemble those presented for Zn²⁺ binding (cf. Fig. 3 of Ref. 17) with low- and high-affinity binding sites of 140 and 50 nmoles of lead per milligram of protein, respectively. The presence of sucrose retards the binding of lead, and considerably less lead is taken up by mitochondria from an acetate medium than from chloride or nitrate media in the absence of energy (Fig. 1). In the presence of phosphate virtually no lead is available to interact with the mitochondrion (4, 6).

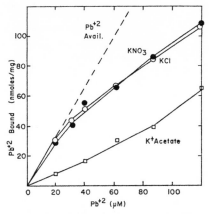

Fig. 1. Passive binding of lead by isolated heart mitochondria. Mitochondria (5 mg of protein) were treated with rotenone and incubated at 25° in 8 ml of the indicated medium (100 mм) containing Tris buffer at pH 7.0. Swelling was monitored by absorbance decrease at 546 mμ for 3 min (cf Fig. 5) and the mitochondria were removed by rapid centrifugation (Sorvall SE-20 rotor: 2 min at 20,000 rpm). The uptake of lead was determined by atomic-absorption spectroscopy of the resulting supernatant fluids.

Energy-dependent increases in lead uptake. The presence of ascorbate-TMPD respiration markedly increases the amount of Pb²⁺ bound by mitochondria suspended in 100 mм K⁺ acetate. Mitochondria isolated under these conditions contain approximately the same amount of Pb²⁺ as that shown for KCl and KNO₃ in Fig. 1. Addition of an uncoupler or inhibitor of respiration abolishes this increment in Pb²⁺ uptake, so that the passive binding curve shown in Fig. 1 for acetate is obtained. Increasing the pH of the suspending medium results in more passive binding of Pb²⁺ from an acetate medium so that the active and passive binding curves converge at pH 8.

The uptake and loss of Pb²⁺ from the acetate medium as a function of the energy status of the mitochondrion can be demonstrated directly using the murexide procedure (Fig. 2). In these experiments mitochondria were deenergized by treatment with rotenone and oligomycin and then treated with Pb²⁺. The murexide indicated passive binding of Pb²⁺ under these conditions to

135

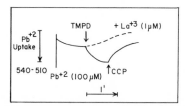

FIG. 2. Respiration-dependent uptake of Pb²⁺ from a medium of K⁺ acetate. Mitochondria (10 mg of protein) were treated with rotenone (1.6 µg/mg) and oligomycin (2 µg/mg) and suspended in 10 ml of a medium of K⁺ acetate (100 mM) and Tris acetate (2 mM, pH 7.1) at 25° in the chamber of an Aminco–Chance spectrometer (12). Murexide (20 µM) was added followed by Pb²⁺ acetate (100 µM), and the absorbance at 540–510 mµ was recorded. Where indicated K⁺ ascorbate (1 mM) and TMPD (40 µM) were added. The dashed trace shows the response in the presence of 1 µM La³⁺. CCP was added to 5 × 10⁻⁷ M where shown.

the same extent as estimation by centrifugation and atomic absorption. When respiration is initiated under these conditions by addition of ascorbate and TMPD, the murexide trace indicates a rapid decrease in free Pb²⁺ in solution (Fig. 2). This uptake is prevented by CCP and if CCP is added after the energy-dependent Pb²⁺ uptake has occurred, the murexide indicates that about the same amount of Pb²⁺ is released from the mitochondria (Fig. 2). The energy-dependent increment in Pb²⁺ uptake is also abolished by 1 µM La³⁺ (Fig. 2). It should be noted that La³⁺ interferes with the passive binding of Pb²⁺ to only a very limited extent at a concentration of 10 µM and does not inhibit passive Pb²⁺ binding at the 1 µM level. ·

Effect of lead on the bromthymol blue response. In contrast to these results with an acetate medium, the amount of lead bound by mitochondria suspended in a medium of KCl or sucrose–KCl does not change significantly as a function of the presence or absence of energy. Indications of an energy-dependent movement of lead analogous to that of Ca²⁺ (13–15) can be seen under these conditions using the membrane-bound pH indicator bromthymol blue (13–15), however. Lead produces an energy-dependent alkalization of this indicator which closely resembles the response to Ca²⁺ (Fig. 3).

The apparent alkalization requires a sustained energy source, such as oxidation of ascorbate–TMPD, and is reversed by addition of uncouplers or a permeant anion such as acetate. Addition of Ca²⁺ prior to the Pb²⁺, reduces the alkalization due to Pb²⁺ and addition of Pb²⁺ before Ca²⁺ results in inhibition of the normal response to Ca²⁺ (Fig. 3). In the presence of succinate respiration, addition of Pb²⁺ results in an initial alkalization which is followed by a spontaneous reversal. This acidification appears to be associated with the loss of capacity to utilize succinate as a source of energy in the presence of Pb²⁺, a response which will be discussed in a subsequent section. Addition of Pb²⁺ rapidly reverses the alkaline shift which follows addition of Ca²⁺ under these conditions, as well. The bromthymol blue alkalization which results from the addition of Pb²⁺ is inhibited by La³⁺, and the inhibition can be overcome by addition of larger amounts of Pb²⁺ (traces not shown). The inhibition of energy-linked Ca²⁺ uptake by added Pb²⁺ can also be demonstrated directly when the uptake of Ca²⁺ from the medium is measured by the atomic-absorption technique.

Induction of passive osmotic swelling in KCl by lead ions. Passive swelling in a medium of KCl requires that the membrane of the mitochondrion be permeable to both K⁺ and Cl⁻ (18, 19). In the absence of inducing agents and a source of energy the mitochondrion does not show appreciable permeability to either of these ions. Previous studies have shown that increasing amounts of an organic mercurial such as CMB will induce a passive permeability to KCl which results in osmotic swelling (20). A similar effect is seen when a suspension of heart mitochondria in 100 mM KCl is titrated with Pb²⁺ (Fig. 4). Considerably higher concentrations of Pb²⁺ than CMB are required to obtain the maximum change in permeability and the resulting ion uptake and swelling. Removal of the Pb²⁺ can be accomplished by addition of an excess of EDTA and, after this removal, respiration-dependent ion extrusion and contraction can be demonstrated (Fig. 4). This reaction closely resembles that seen after removal of CMB with excess thiol reagents (cf. Ref. 20). Lead-induced swelling in KCl occurs with lower levels of lead when

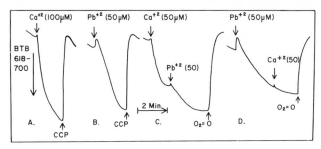

Fig. 3. Respiration-dependent changes in bromthymol blue absorbance as a function of Ca^{2+} and Pb^{2+} addition. Mitochondria (10 mg of protein) were treated with rotenone and suspended in 10 ml of a medium of sucrose (100 mM), KCl (10 mM), and Tris–Cl (2 mM, pH 7.1), containing Tris ascorbate (2 mM) and TMPD (0.4 mM). Changes in absorbance of bromthymol blue (3.0 μM) were followed at 618–700 mμ in the Aminco–Chance. Where indicated Ca^{2+} (50 or 100 μM) and Pb^{2+} (50 μM) were added. A simultaneous record of O_2 uptake (not reproduced) showed the anaerobic point. The concentration of CCP was 5×10^{-7} M added as indicated.

the permeability to Cl^- is increased by raising the pH to 8.0.

Titration of beef heart mitochondria suspended in 100 mM KNO_3 shows that a given amount of bound Pb^{2+} is more effective in inducing swelling in this medium than in the KCl medium as just described (Fig. 5). Since mitochondria are much more permeable to NO_3^- than to Cl^- at neutral pH (9), this result can be taken to mean that lower levels of bound Pb^{2+} are required to induce passive permeability to K^+ than to K^+ and Cl^-. This interpretation is supported by the observation that valinomycin-treated mitochondria (which are permeable to K^+) show almost the same swelling increment in the presence of bound Pb^{2+} as do mitochondria in the absence of the ionophore. The induction of permeability to K^+ by Pb^{2+} at moderate levels of binding is also supported by the fact that a given amount of Pb^{2+} will induce more swelling in the presence of CMS, a reagent known to increase passive permeability to Cl^- (21). It seems, therefore, that Pb^{2+} first induces an increased permeability to K^+ and, as more Pb^{2+} interacts with the membrane, an increased permeability to Cl^- is also induced. The alteration in permeability is not specific for K^+, since the binding of 60–70 nmoles of Pb^{2+} per milligram of protein to heart mitochondria results in passive osmotic swelling in NH_4^+, Li^+, and Na^+ ni-

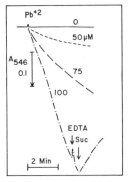

Fig. 4. Induction of passive osmotic swelling in KCl by Pb^{2+}. Mitochondria (5 mg of protein) were treated with rotenone and suspended at 25° in 8 ml of KCl (100 mM) and Tris–Cl (2 mM, pH 7). Swelling was initiated by addition of the indicated amount of $PbCl_2$ and was monitored by recording the absorbance at 546 mμ. EDTA (1 mM) and succinate (2 mM) were added where indicated to initiate the respiration-dependent contraction.

trates as well as in KNO_3. Swelling in tetramethyl ammonium nitrate is not induced by this level of Pb^{2+}, however, so some measure of selective permeability to cations is retained by the Pb^{2+}-treated membrane.

Activation by lead of respiration-dependent accumulation of K^+ and acetate. Beef heart mitochondria suspended in K^+ acetate or

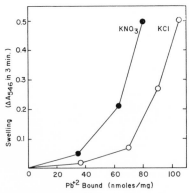

FIG. 5. Passive swelling in KNO₃ and KCl as a function of bound Pb²⁺. Passive swelling and the amount of Pb²⁺ bound were determined as described in Fig. 1.

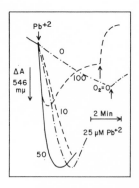

FIG. 6. Activation by Pb²⁺ of the respiration-dependent accumulation of K⁺ acetate. Mitochondria (5 mg of protein) were treated with rotenone and suspended in 10 ml of a medium of sucrose (100 mM), K⁺ acetate (10 mM), and Tris acetate (2 mM, pH 7.0) containing Tris ascorbate (2 mM) and TMPD (0.4 mM). The respiration-dependent uptake of K⁺ and acetate and the resulting osmotic swelling were followed by the decrease in absorbance at 546 mμ in the Eppendorf photometer. Pb²⁺ acetate at 10, 25, 50, or 100 μM was added as shown.

sucrose plus K⁺ acetate spontaneously accumulate ions and swell osmotically by a respiration-dependent reaction (10, 19). The study shown in Fig. 6 establishes that low concentrations of Pb²⁺ markedly activate this reaction when the mitochondria are respiring with ascorbate–TMPD. The study shown was carried out in 100 mM sucrose containing 10 mM K⁺ acetate. In this medium the accumulation of ions is prevented and reversed (due to sucrose osmotic pressure) by uncouplers and by inhibitors of respiration. The increased increment in swelling and ion uptake which occurs in the presence of Pb²⁺ is also sensitive to uncouplers and inhibitors and depends on the amount of Pb²⁺ added (Fig. 6). Higher concentrations of Pb²⁺ induce a biphasic reaction with a rapid swelling phase followed by a passive contraction and, finally, by a rapid contraction at anaerobiosis (Fig. 6). Similar activation of respiration-dependent accumulation of K⁺ and acetate has been reported in the presence of Zn²⁺, Cd²⁺, and mercurial reagents (10, 20–23). The contraction which occurs at anaerobiosis or on addition of CCP is much more rapid in lead-treated mitochondria than that seen in the absence of lead (Fig. 6), a result consistent with an increased passive permeability to K⁺ in the lead-treated membrane.

Release of endogenous K⁺ by lead. Another line of experimentation which indicates that an increased permeability to K⁺ is induced by lead is summarized in Fig. 7. Addition of increasing amounts of lead to mitochondria respiring with endogenous substrates in a K⁺-free medium results in a greatly accelerated loss of endogenous K⁺ (Fig. 7A). There is an immediate appearance of H⁺ in the medium upon addition of lead which is due principally to the acidity of the lead nitrate added. After this pH shift, an uptake of H⁺ from the medium is observed which roughly parallels the K⁺ loss. In the presence of an uncoupler or a respiratory inhibitor there is an apparent discharge of a pH gradient from the mitochondria and very much less tendency to release K⁺ and take up H⁺ is then observed as a result of lead addition (Fig. 7B).

Effects of lead on respiration. The effects of lead on mitochondrial respiration vary considerably with the experimental conditions employed. One of the factors to be considered is the intrinsic sensitivity of the enzyme systems involved to inhibition by the heavy metal. For example, titration of suc-

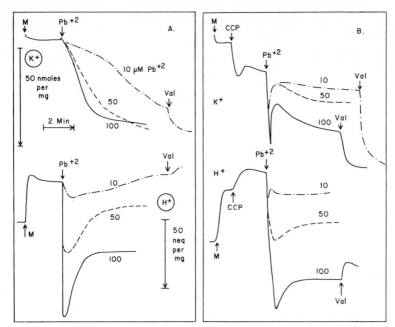

FIG. 7. Pb²⁺-dependent release of endogenous K⁺ from beef heart mitochondria in the presence of endogenous respiration (A) and of uncoupler (B). Mitochondria (10 mg of protein) were added to 10 ml of a medium of tetramethylammonium chloride (100 mM) containing Tris–Cl (2 mM, pH 7.3) and the H⁺ and K⁺ content monitored with the appropriate glass electrodes using a common reference electrode. In part A, Pb²⁺ was added in the presence of endogenous respiration to 10, 50, or 100 μM as indicated. In part B the mitochondria were uncoupled with CCP (5 × 10⁻⁷ M), and the titration was repeated. Valinomycin was added to 2 × 10⁻⁷ M where indicated.

cinate respiration of submitochondrial particles in a KCl medium with lead (Fig. 8) shows that oxidation of this substrate is considerably more sensitive to Pb²⁺ than is the oxidation of DPNH by these particles. Succinoxidase is inhibited 50 % by the presence of 10 nmoles/mg of Pb²⁺ (which is bound almost quantitatively by the particles under these conditions) whereas 80 nmoles of Pb²⁺ per milligram are required to produce the corresponding reduction in DPNH oxidation. As with the intact mitochondria, less of the available Pb²⁺ is bound by the submitochondrial particles in a medium of K⁺ acetate (100 mM) and the amount of added Pb²⁺ necessary for 50 % inhibition of succinoxidase increases to about 30 nmoles/mg.

The oxidation of ascorbate–TMPD by submitochondrial particles is not affected by addition of even high levels of Pb²⁺ (more than 300 nmoles/mg of protein). The inhibition of succinoxidase activity by Pb²⁺ and the inhibition of succinic dehydrogenase activity (as measured by the use of phenazine methosulfate as acceptor) show virtually superimposable titration curves in these particles. These results suggest that the primary site of inhibition of succinoxidase activity by Pb²⁺ is the succinic dehydrogenase step. In further support of this suggestion is the observation that cytochrome *b* (as measured by 430- to 490-mμ absorbance changes) shifts to a more oxidized steady state after addition of Pb²⁺ in the presence of succinate.

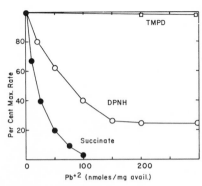

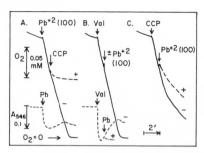

FIG. 8. Inhibition of succinate and DPNH oxidation in submitochondrial particles by Pb^{2+}. Particles (10 mg of protein) were added to 10 ml of a medium of KCl (100 mM) and Tris–Cl (2 mM, pH 7.1), treated with the indicated amount of Pb^{2+} and respiration initiated by the addition of either K^+ succinate (2 mM) or DPNH (1 mM). The initial uninhibited rates were 0.25 μatoms O_2 per minute per milligram for DPNH and 0.13 for succinate.

FIG. 9. Effects of lead on respiration and swelling with glutamate plus malate. Heart mitochondria (1 mg/ml) were suspended in KCl (100 mM) containing 2 mM Tris–Cl (pH 7) and glutamate plus malate (2 mM each) as substrate. Where indicated 100 μM lead nitrate (100 nmoles/mg), CCP (5×10^{-7} M), or valinomycin (2×10^{-7} M) were added, and the rate of respiration and the absorbance at 546 mμ were recorded.

A. Effects of lead on DPNH-linked respiration. In addition to the intrinsic sensitivity of the respiratory enzymes to lead, a number of other factors appear to be able to affect the respiration of intact mitochondria in the presence of this metal ion. For example, with TMPD–ascorbate as substrate, lead activation of ion transport (Fig. 6), combined with the relative insensitivity of this respiration to the heavy metal, result in marked activation of respiration. A similar situation has been observed with the more physiological substrate combination of glutamate plus malate (Fig. 9). Heart mitochondria respiring with this pair of substrates in a KCl medium show nearly as great an activation in oxidation rate after addition of 100 μM lead as is seen with valinomycin under these conditions. The lead-dependent elevated rate of respiration is extremely sensitive to inhibition by an uncoupler such as CCP (Fig. 9A). In the KCl medium there is a small cycle of swelling and contraction after the addition of lead which closely resembles that seen with valinomycin under these conditions (Fig. 9A vs 9B, and Ref. 24). In a sucrose–K$^+$ acetate medium, lead produces activation of respiration and large-amplitude swelling

cycles in the presence of this substrate pair. Lead does not inhibit the elevated rate of respiration produced by valinomycin when glutamate plus malate are oxidized (Fig. 9B), so it must be concluded that the inherent sensitivity to lead of the enzymes carrying out the respiration is low. Lead does inhibit the respiration elicited by an uncoupler under these conditions, however (Fig. 9C), but it should be noted that the opposite order of addition (Pb^{2+} followed by CCP, Fig. 9A) is much more inhibitory. Lead, like valinomycin, produces higher rates of respiration in the presence of K^+ than when a suspending medium of NaCl or tetramethylammonium chloride is used in place of KCl. The major effect of lead on glutamate–malate oxidation, therefore, seems to be associated with increased uptake of K^+ and the energy expenditure associated with ion movements, rather than heavy-metal inhibition of respiration.

Respiration with pyruvate plus malate in a KCl medium is activated briefly by lead at low concentrations, and some swelling is associated with these brief bursts of respiration. The oxygen uptake rapidly declines under these conditions, however. The elevated rates of respiration activated by uncouplers and by valinomycin are very sensitive to inhibition by lead (2.5 μM lead

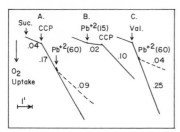

Fig. 10. Effects of lead on respiration of beef heart mitochondria with succinate. The experimental conditions were identical to those of Fig. 9 except that succinate (2 mM) was the substrate and 5 mg of mitochondria were suspended in 10 ml of the KCl medium. The rate of respiration in μatoms O_2 per minute per milligram is indicated after each addition. The concentration of lead (nmoles per milligram) is given in parentheses.

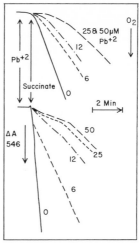

Fig. 11. Inhibition by Pb^{2+} of the succinate-dependent accumulation of K^+ acetate. Mitochondria were suspended in a medium of K^+ acetate (100 mM) under the conditions described in Fig. 10. The effect of increasing concentrations of Pb^{2+} on the swelling and respiration supported by 2 mM K^+ succinate is shown.

inhibits both rates by about 50% under the conditions of Fig. 9, using 2 mM pyruvate in place of glutamate). This response is consistent with the known sensitivity of the pyruvic dehydrogenase complex to heavy metals.

Oxidation of β-hydroxybutyrate in the presence of lead falls between the extremes just discussed for glutamate (rather insensitive) and pyruvate (sensitive at low levels of lead). The uncoupler-activated and the valinomycinactivated rates are both inhibited about 50% by 25 mM lead in a KCl medium. This amount of lead activates the State 4 (25) rate from 2- to 3-fold, but again where significant swelling appears, the activated rate declines rapidly.

B. Effects of lead on succinate respiration. Addition of lead to intact mitochondria respiring with succinate invariably results in a decreased rate of oxidation, but the relative response to a given amount of added lead depends on the energy status of the mitochondrion and on the medium employed. In a KCl medium, for example, the uncoupled rate of respiration is inhibited 50% by addition of 50–60 nmoles of lead per milligram of protein, but the lower State 4 rate requires only 15 nmoles/mg for 50% inhibition (Fig. 10). This results in an apparent activation of respiration by added uncoupler at concentrations of lead in this region (Fig. 10B). Lead is clearly inhibitory to the CCP-

induced rate when the opposite order of addition is employed (Fig. 10A). It appears likely that lead is moving toward the matrix under these conditions (cf Fig. 3 results), and the internal concentration of heavy metal may be elevated by this energy-dependent uptake in the absence of an uncoupler and hence cause inhibition at a lower nominal concentration. The high rates of succinate respiration elicited by valinomycin are inhibited by lead at rather low levels (10 nmoles of lead per milligram protein for 50% inhibition; Fig. 10C).

In an acetate medium the succinate-supported accumulation of ions and osmotic swelling (10, 19) is strongly inhibited by addition of lead (Fig. 11). Since the respiration and swelling curves are not linear, it is difficult to compare the relative efficiencies of swelling supported by succinate in each case, but it appears that the lead-insensitive respiration supports less swelling than does respiration in the absence of this inhibitor.

An additional factor to consider in evaluating the effects of lead on succinate-sup-

TABLE I

EFFECT OF LEAD ON EXCHANGE AND RETENTION OF ^{14}C-LABELED SUCCINATE BY HEART MITOCHONDRIA[a]

	No unlabeled succinate added			Labeled succinate retained	Succinate (1 mM) added supernatant	Increase due to exchange	Exchange
	Residue	Sup.	Tot				
	(cpm)			(% Control)	(cpm)	(cpm)	(%)
Control	3370	1425	4795	100	2660	1235	37
CMS (100 μM)	2950	1530	4480	85	1955	425	14
Pb²⁺ (5 μM)	3540	1460	5000	100	2260	800	23
Pb²⁺ (50 μM)	2420	2620	5040	71	4250	1630	67

[a] Mitochondria were treated with rotenone and antimycin labeled with [14C]-succinate as described by Robinson and Williams (33), and incubated at 5 mg/ml in a medium of KCl (100 mM), Tris–Cl (2 mM, pH 7.1). CMS or Pb²⁺ was added to the indicated concentration, and the incubation at 0° was continued for 1 min. Succinate was added to a concentration of 1 mM to half the flasks, the incubation was continued for 2 min, and the mitochondria were removed by rapid centrifugation (Sorvall SE-12 rotor operated at 20,000 rpm for 4 min). The radioactivity of the supernatant fluids and residues was then compared as described (33).

ported respiration and reactions dependent on this oxidation, is the ability of lead to interfere with the uptake and retention of succinate (Table I). It is apparent that lower levels of lead (5 μM) interfere with succinate exchange across the membrane in much the same way as CMS (percentage of exchange decreases from 37 to 23 %), but as the amount of lead is increased, the ability of the mitochondrion to retain succinate is diminished (71 % of control radioactivity retained in the absence of exchange against unlabeled succinate).

DISCUSSION

The present studies have established that lead is bound avidly by isolated heart mitocondria and that the amount of binding will depend on the anionic composition of the suspending medium. It is also established that lead, like a number of other divalent cations, is transported by the mitochondrion in an energy-requiring reaction. The ability of lead to inhibit the uptake of Ca²⁺ and the sensitivity of the respiration-dependent lead uptake to La³⁺ suggest that the heavy metal may utilize the Ca²⁺ carrier system of the mitochondrion (13, 26) in its movements. The interaction of lead with the mitochondrial membrane results in increased permeability to such cations as K⁺, and at higher levels of lead the permeability to anions is increased as well. This increased permeability

is reflected under the appropriate conditions in (a) passive osmotic swelling (Fig. 4), (b) activated energy-dependent ion accumulation (Fig. 6), and (c) increased loss of endogenous and accumulated ions (Figs. 6 and 7).

The high affinity of lead for phosphate and for thiols suggests that these groups may be involved in the binding of lead by the mitochondrion, but attempts to define specific sites of lead interaction in terms of specific responses have not been encouraging. Net uptake of lead is not decreased by prior interaction of mitochondria or submitochondrial particles with CMS or other thiol-group reagents. The murexide procedure shows that these reagents do decrease the rate of uptake of lead, however, and it, therefore, appears that at least a portion of the heavy-metal binding may involve thiols. As has been noted for Zn²⁺ (17), the removal of phospholipids by extraction has little effect on the binding of lead seen at lower concentrations but results in decreased binding as the lead concentration is increased (cf. Ref. 17, Fig. 8 for the analogous curves for Zn²⁺ uptake). The evidence at hand suggests that a variety of binding sites are available for lead uptake by the membrane.

The effects of lead on respiration in vitro vary considerably and depend on which substrate is used, the suspending medium, order of addition, and the metabolic state of the mitochondria. The present studies suggest that the observed effect of lead on respiration represents an interplay between (a) the intrinsic ability of lead to inhibit the enzymes involved, (b) the amount of lead available to interact with these enzymes, (c) the amount of energy-linked ion transport which is activated by lead, (d) active movements of lead itself, and (e) effects of lead on substrate uptake and retention.

In the case of ascorbate–TMPD oxidation the enzymes show no inhibition by lead, and when uptake of ions is activated as a result of the heavy metal-induced change in permeability, the response seen is a marked activation of respiration. Respiration with glutamate and malate shows a similar effect. With these substrates the response to lead is similar to that to valinomycin. Succinate oxidation is more sensitive to lead than is DPNH oxidation in submitochondrial particles, but in intact mitochondria succinoxidase activity in the presence of lead depends on the metabolic state. Succinate oxidation is less sensitive to lead in uncoupled mitochondria and it appears possible that respiration-dependent uptake of lead may increase the concentration of inhibitor on the matrix side of the membrane in coupled mitochondria. This would lead to strongly inhibited State 4 respiration which could be relieved to some extent by addition of an uncoupler. This suggestion is analogous to that advanced by Mitchell (27) to explain site-specific uncoupling by guanidine derivatives and by Palmeri and Klingenberg (28) for azide inhibition. The contribution of the effects of lead on substrate transport (cf 29 for a review) to the observed effects on respiration is not clear, although the present study has shown an increased loss of endogenous succinate in the presence of lead (Table I) and Krall *et al.* (7) have shown a 20–30% decrease in both pyruvate and succinate exchange in kidney mitochondria from lead-treated rats.

It would appear that direct evaluation of oxidative phosphorylation as a measure of coupling in lead-treated mitochondria (2, 3, 7) would be difficult to interpret, since addition of even low levels of P_i has resulted in reversal of many of the lead-dependent effects reported here. In agreement with previous reports (4, 6) we can conclude that the level of P_i in the medium can be the overriding factor in determining the response of the mitochondrion to lead *in vitro*. For this reason it is difficult to specify which of the phenomena described here might contribute to the observed deterioration of mitochondria after lead ingestion *in vivo* (cf 1, 2). Early studies with isotopic lead (30) indicate that lead reaches all major subcellular fractions of liver and kidney *in vivo*. It is, therefore, quite possible that many of the effects described here may be of physiological importance and also that changes in permeability similar to those described for heart mitochondria in the present work may contribute to the observed effects of lead on erythrocytes, capillaries, and other membrane systems (cf 31 for a recent review). It would also seem possible that a number of well-established antagonistic effects of lead and Ca^{2+} (see Ref. 32, for example) might be explained by the ability of lead to interact with Ca^{2+}-binding proteins in analogy to the mitochondrial transport system.

ACKNOWLEDGMENTS

These studies were supported in part by United States Public Health Service Grant HE 09364 and by a Grant-in-Aid from the American Heart Association. For the previous communication in this series see Ref. 10. A preliminary report of a portion of this work has been made (5).

REFERENCES

1. GOYER, R. A., *Lab. Invest.* **19,** 71 (1968).
2. GOYER, R. A., KRALL, A., AND KIMBALL, J. P., *Lab. Invest.* **19,** 78 (1968).
3. GOYER, R. A. AND KRALL, R., *J. Cell. Biol.* **41,** 393 (1969).
4. KOEPPE, D. E. AND MILLER, R. J., *Science* **167,** 1376 (1970).
5. BRIERLEY, G. P., SCOTT, K. M., HWANG, K. M., AND JURKOWITZ, M., *Fed. Proc.* **30,** 1285A (1971).
6. CARDONA, E., LESSLER, M. A., AND BRIERLEY, G. P., *Proc. Soc. Exp. Biol. Med.* **136,** 300 (1971).
7. KRALL, A. R., MENG, T. T., HARMON, S. J., AND DOUGHERTY, W. J., *Fed. Proc.* **30,** 1285A (1971).
8. SETTLEMIRE, C. T., HUNTER, G. R., AND BRIERLEY, G. P., *Biochim. Biophys. Acta* **162,** 487 (1968).

9. Brierley, G. P., Jurkowitz, M., Scott, K. M., and Merola, A. J., *J. Biol. Chem.* **245**, 5404 (1970).
10. Brierley, G. P., Jurkowitz, M., Scott, K. M., and Merola, A. J., *Arch. Biochem. Biophys.* in press.
11. Hunter, G. R., and Brierley, G. P., *Biochim. Biophys. Acta* **180**, 68 (1969).
12. Merola, A. J., Scott, K. M., and Brierley, G. P., *Anal. Biochem.* **41**, 455 (1971).
13. Mela, L., *Biochemistry* **8**, 2481 (1969).
14. Chance, B., and Mela, L., *Biochemistry* **5**, 3220 (1966).
15. Ghosh, A. K., and Chance, B., *Arch. Biochem. Biophys.* **138**, 483 (1970).
16. King, T. E., *Methods Enzymol.* **10**, 322 (1967).
17. Jacobus, W. E., and Brierley, G. P., *J. Biol. Chem.* **244**, 4995 (1969).
18. Chappell, J. B., and Crofts, A. R., in "Regulation of Metabolic Processes in Mitochondria" (J. M. Tager, S. Popa, E. Quagliariello, and E. C. Slater, eds.), p. 293. Elsevier, New York, 1966.
19. Brierley, G. P., Settlemire, C. T., and Knight, V. A., *Arch. Biochem. Biophys.* **126**, 276 (1968).
20. Scott, K. M., Knight, V. A., Settlemire, C. T., and Brierley, G. P., *Biochemistry* **9**, 714 (1970).
21. Brierley, G. P., Scott, K. M., and Jurkowitz, M., *J. Biol. Chem.* **246**, 2241 (1971).
22. Brierley, G. P. and Settlemire, C. T., *J. Biol. Chem.* **242**, 4324 (1967).
23. Brierley, G. P., Knight, V. A., and Settlemire, C. T., *J. Biol. Chem.* **243**, 5035 (1968).
24. Brierley, G. P., *Biochemistry* **9**, 697 (1970).
25. Chance, B., and Williams, G. R., *J. Biol. Chem.* **217**, 383 (1955).
26. Lehninger, A. L., *Biochem. Biophys. Res. Commun.* **42**, 312 (1971).
27. Mitchell, P., "Chemiosmotic Coupling in Oxidative and Photosynthetic Phosphorylation," Glynn Research, Ltd., Bodmin, Cornwall, 1966.
28. Palmeri, F., and Klingenberg, M., *Eur. J. Biochem.* **1**, 439 (1967).
29. Chappell, J. B., *Brit. Med. Bull.* **24**, 150 (1968).
30. Lang, H. and Fingerhut, M., *Arch. Exp. Pathol. Pharmakol.* **235**, 41 (1958).
31. Hammond, P. B., in "Essays in Toxicology" (F. R. Blood, ed.), Vol. I, p. 115. Academic Press, New York, 1969.
32. Six, K. M., and Goyer, R. A., *J. Lab. Clin. Med.* **76**, 933 (1970).
33. Robinson, B., and Williams, G. R., *Biochim. Biophys. Acta* **216**, 63 (1970).

Comparison of Delta-Aminolevulinic Acid Levels in Urine and Blood Lead Levels for Screening Children for Lead Poisoning

Thomas Murphy, B.A. and Martha L. Lepow, M.D.

A variety of methods have been used to detect increased body burdens of lead in young children and especially to find those children at risk for lead encephalopathy. Two of these methods have been utilized extensively during the past few years for mass screening: the determination of blood lead levels[1] and the measurement of urinary delta-aminolevulinic acid.[2]

This report presents a review of the literature concerning these two procedures and the results obtained by the authors in a comparative study of the two methods.

Any screening procedure for increased exposure to lead should have statistical validity and an economical method of analysis. Additionally, it should involve a sample that is easy to collect and store. Although there are several different methods of lead analysis, they all share in common a serious limitation: the requirement of a venipuncture to obtain a blood sample of 2-12 cc.

More recently the measurement of urinary delta-aminolevulinic acid (ALA) has been utilized in screening for increased body burden of lead to circumvent the problem of obtaining samples of venous blood. The rationale for this test is based on the effect of an increased body burden of lead on heme synthesis. By binding sulfhydryl groups, lead causes inhibition of ALA dehydratase, the enzyme which condenses two molecules of ALA to form porphobilinogen. The result of this inhibition is an increase in the quantity of ALA in the blood followed by an increase of ALA in the urine. Selander and co-workers have shown that among industrial workers with symptoms of lead poisoning a definite correlation exists between blood lead levels and the quantity of ALA in the urine.[3]

These same investigators have also shown that blood lead levels decreased faster than ALA excretion among asymptomatic workers with interrupted exposure to a heavily leaded environment.[4] Thus, the relationship between the two values is not always linear.

Several studies have been carried out in children in which random blood lead levels and urinary ALA levels have been compared. Davis reported that the incidence of negative urinary ALA tests was only 4% when blood lead concentration was higher than 50 μgm/100 ml, the upper limit of normal.[2] Vincent and Ullman studied 57 children by both methods and found no children with blood lead levels greater than 50 μgm/100 ml* with a negative urinary ALA test.[5]

In contrast with the reports of these investigators are the data of Blanksma[6] and Hull[7] and their co-workers. Both groups reported essentially no correlation between the two determinations. In both studies, there was a large number of children with blood lead levels in the range in which chelation therapy would be required who had negative urinary ALA tests. On the other hand, both investigators showed that most subjects with positive urine ALA tests had low blood levels on subsequent testing. Due to conflicting data in the literature, the following study was undertaken to obtain comparative data on the two tests as performed in local laboratories. The study was part of a large screening program using urinary ALA measurement among children in low income areas in Hartford, Connecticut.

Study Population

Seventy-six Spanish-speaking and black children ages 1-4 from "high risk" areas were included. All of these children lived in housing composed of multiple dwelling units built before 1940.

Included were children who were being checked one year after a previous evaluation for increased body burden of lead; children who required a blood lead level determination as a result of a positive ALA test discovered during the screening program; and a few children who were tested during a visit to a sick-child clinic. None of these subjects had symptoms of lead intoxication. Single blood and urine samples were obtained simultaneously. Urine samples were collected in glass bottles with preservative, wrapped to protect them from sunlight, and placed in a cooler. ALA determinations were performed by the Connecticut State Health Department according to the Sun Method[5] modified by Vincent and Ullman.[9] Blood samples were obtained with lead-free syringes and frozen in lead-free heparinized tubes until analyzed. All blood lead analyses were carried out by one of the authors using the method of Selander and Cramer[10] modified by F. W. Sunderman, Jr.[11] Normal blood lead levels are considered to be less than 50 μgm/100 ml of whole blood and normal urine ALA concentration less than 0.55 mgm/100 ml.

Results

The comparison of blood lead and urinary ALA levels on specimens obtained simultaneously is shown in Figure 1. Of the 76 children tested, 48 were found to have normal blood lead levels and normal urinary ALA levels. Eighteen children had elevated ALA levels with normal blood lead levels. Five children had both elevated blood lead and urinary ALA levels and finally, five children had elevated blood lead levels with normal urinary

ALA content. Three of the 5 with elevated blood lead levels and negative ALA tests had been found to have had an elevated ALA test 1-4 months previously.

These data indicate an incidence of "false positives" of 78% and an incidence of "false negatives" of 50%.

Discussion

These results paralleled those of Blanksma and Hull. "False negative" results may be caused by one of several factors. In a randomly obtained urine sample, there may be problems of concentration. It would be of considerable interest to determine urinary ALA on each sample of urine excreted during a 24 hour period, since it is likely that there is considerable variation in ALA concentration. Since ALA is labile in light, heat, and in alkaline solution, specimens must be carefully handled. In spite of precautions taken to avoid obvious pitfalls, it is difficult to be entirely certain that some false negative results might not have occurred as a result of improper handling of specimens.

Another disturbing feature was the observation that many children who had had an abnormal ALA test had a normal blood lead level. This led to the development of an hypothesis: that perhaps children with an increased body burden of metabolically active lead stored in tissue may manifest a positive urinary ALA test without an elevated blood lead level. This postulate is currently being tested by giving challenges with single doses of EDTA according to the method of Whitaker[12] except that the urinary output of lead is monitored over an eight hour period instead of 24 hours.

Data obtained in this manner in three children with positive urinary ALA tests and blood lead levels of less than 40 μgms/100 ml indicated that two of the three excreted over 990 μgms of lead in eight hours. In accordance with Whitaker's data,

SIMULTANEOUS COMPARISON OF BLOOD LEAD AND URINE ALA TESTS IN 77 SUBJECTS (one to four year olds)

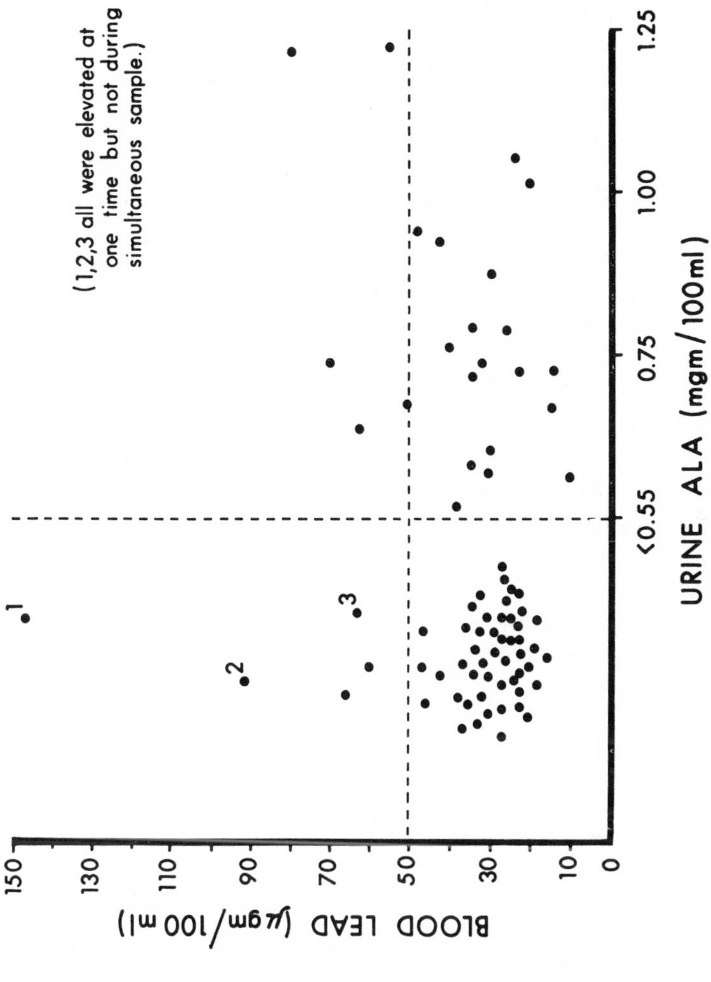

(1,2,3 all were elevated at one time but not during simultaneous sample.)

Figure 1

these values indicate markedly increased body burdens of lead.

It is not known whether those three children were still eating leaded paint and it is also not known whether these results will be confirmed in a larger study now underway.

Another factor to be considered is the possibility that intermittent ingestion may be the rule rather than the exception among children with pica for paint. If this is the case, results observed in the present study could be compared with results obtained by Cramer and Selander in their studies of industrial workers with intermittent exposure. Although blood lead levels might be low, urinary ALA excretion would continue at abnormal levels. Since the method of ALA determination also measures aminoacetones, it may be that some of the false positives are due to those substances rather than ALA. As for those children with blood lead levels above 60 μgms/100 ml and normal urinary ALA, it is possible that the duration of exposure has been very short and very recent.

It is evident that in children, as in industrial workers, the blood lead level and urinary ALA concentration cannot be used interchangeably. Blood lead will be elevated in acute intoxication or in continual chronic ingestion when the tissue capacity for storage is exceeded, whereas ALA may be elevated in chronic and/or intermittent ingestion and possibly for some time after ingestion has ceased. The results of versene challenges suggest that some children with positive urinary ALA tests with normal blood lead levels may have an excessive amount of stored lead in their body tissues. More data are required to confirm this postulate.

Although surveys using random urine samples in which ALA is measured may identify children who have had excessive lead intake, that test alone cannot be depended upon for identifying a child who requires chelation therapy to prevent encephalopathy.

Thus, all such children should have a blood lead determination performed. In order to detect children with blood lead levels of 60 μgms whose ALA test might be negative, continuous monitoring of blood lead levels must be carried out. Another possible mechanism for discovering that group of children before they become symptomatic would be to measure the inhibition of ALA dehydratase by lead directly in the red cells. This might be done on a small sample of blood. Hernberg[12] reports a close negative correlation between the enzyme levels and blood lead levels. At blood levels of 40 μgms, the enzyme is 50% inhibited and at blood levels of approximately 70 μgm/100 ml, the enzyme is 90% inhibited. This places some limitation on the test as a screening device for identifying children who require immediate treatment since the test loses its ability to discriminate varying increments in lead levels from 70-200 μgm. Nonetheless, if this test were employed for screening purposes, any child with 90% inhibition of enzyme should have a blood lead level determination. Theoretically, the enzyme level should be decreased before there would be an increased concentration of the substrate (ALA) in the blood. Until a micromethod for blood lead determination is forthcoming, measurement of the enzyme might be a valid approach for large scale screening.

Another reason for pursuing the enzyme specifically are the findings of Millar and co-workers who have shown that modest elevations in blood lead in suckling rats results in a reduction in both blood and brain ALA dehydratase activity.[12] Translated to man: if brain dehydratase is inhibited at the same level as blood dehydratase, then children will be "at risk" of incurring central nervous system damage at considerably lower blood lead levels than are now acceptable.

Thus, it might be important to monitor the prevalence of partial inhibition of enzyme to detect individuals who are suffering from increased exposure and establish measures to remove available lead from the environment.

A method for blood lead determinations utilizing atomic absorption spectroscopy but only requiring 10 μl of whole blood is under development.[8] Among 78 samples of blood in which lead levels were determined by the micromethod and compared with results obtained by the standard colorimetric method, the correlation coefficient was 0.989. Thus, although it is experimental and requires costly machinery, the micromethod procedure seems to have considerable promise.

Conclusion

The use of urinary ALA content for screening for lead poisoning in children will not identify a significant percentage of children with elevated blood lead levels who may require treatment. In the present investigation, 50% of the children with elevated blood lead levels had normal ALA content in the urine. Of 23 children with a positive ALA test in the urine, 18 had normal blood lead levels. The results obtained among three children with normal blood lead and elevated ALA levels who were given versene challenges seems to suggest that these are not all false positives since two of the three children subsequently showed an abnormal output of lead in the urine. The data suggest a complimentary role for the two tests. Blood lead determination would be more valuable where recent ingestion is suspected or symptoms of lead intoxication are present while ALA would be valuable in those who are suspected of having increased amounts of stored lead. Such an hypothesis suggests that the use of either test *alone* for screening would result in children at one end or the other of a spectrum not being identified. Any child with a positive ALA test must have a blood lead determination.

Obviously, more data is necessary on the group of "false positives" to, in fact, determine whether or not they comprise a clinically significant group of children who require therapy. Any further comment on the merits of ALA versus blood lead must await the collection of such data.

Measurement of ALA dehydratase is valuable for industrial screening and theoretically should have great value in screening for abnormal lead exposure among young children. The micromethod for determination of blood lead levels is attractive: yet more technical development is required before it will have widespread use. At present measurement of Blood Lead is the most reliable screening tool for detection of childhood lead poisoning.

Since this manuscript was submitted for publication, Weissberg, Lipschutz, and Oski have demonstrated that the measurement of delta-aminolevulinic acid dehydratase activity in a small sample of circulating blood cells is a sensitive method of detecting increased lead burden in young children.[16]

References

1. Blanksma, L., Sachs, H. K., Murray, E. F. and O'Connell, M. J.: "Incidence of High Blood Lead Levels in Chicago Children," *Pediatrics* 44:661, 1969.
2. Davis, J. R. and Andelman, S. L.: "Urinary Delta-aminolevulinic Acid (ALA) Levels in Lead Poisoning. I. A Modified Method for the Rapid Determination of Urinary Delta-aminolevulinic Acid Using Disposable Ion-Exchange Chromatography Columns," *Archives of Environmental Health* 15:53-59, 1967.
3. Selander, S., Cramer, K., and Hallberg, L.: "Studies in Lead Poisoning. Oral Therapy with Penicillamine, Relationship between Lead in Blood and Other Laboratory Tests," *British Journal of Industrial Medicine* 23:282-291, 1966.
4. Selander, S. and Cramer, K.: "Interrelationships between Lead in Blood, Lead in Urine, and ALA in Urine During Lead Work," *British Journal of Industrial Medicine,* 27:28-39, 1970.
5. Vincent, W. and Ullman, W.: Letter to the Editor. *American Journal of Clinical Pathology,* 53:963-964, 1970.
6. Blanksma, L. et al.: "Failure of the Urinary Delta-aminolevulinic Acid Test to Detect Pediatric Lead Poisoning," *American Journal of Clinical Pathology,* 53:956-962, 1970.
7. Hull, H. and Chisolm, J.: Unpublished data.
8. Sun, M. W., Stein, E. and Gruen, F. W.: "A Single Column Method for the Determination of Urinary Delta-aminolevulinic Acid," *Clinical Chemistry,* 15:183-189, 1969.
9. Vincent, W. F. and Ullman, W. W.: "The Preservation of Urine Specimens for Delta-aminolevulinic Acid Determination," *Clinical Chemistry,* 16: 612, 1970.

10. Sunderman, F. W., Jr.: "Measurements of Blood Lead by Atomic Absorption Spectrophotometry," Manual of the Proceedings for the Applied Seminar on Chemical Hematology, 125, 1970 (W. H. Green, St. Louis, in press).

11. Selander, S. and Cramer, K.: "Determination of Lead in Blood by Atomic Absorption Spectrophotometry," *British Journal of Industrial Medicine,* 25:209-213, 1968.

12. Whitaker, J. A., Austin, W. and Nelson, J. D.: "Early Detection of Lead Poisoning, *Pediatrics,* 29:384-388, 1962.

13. Hernberg, S.: "Delta-aminolevulinic Acid Dehydratase as a Measure of Lead Exposure," *Archives of Environmental Health,* 21:140-145, 1970.

14. Millar, J. A. et al.: "Lead and Delta-aminolevulinic Acid Dehydratase Levels in Mentally Retarded Children and in Lead Poisoned Suckling Rats," *Lancet,* 2:695-698, 1970.

15. Delvas, H. T.: "A Microsampling Method for the Rapid Determination of Lead in Blood by A. A. S," *Analyst,* 95:431-438, 1970.

16. Weissberg, J. B., Lipschutz, F. and Oski, Frank A.: "Delta-aminolevulinic Acid Dehydratase Activity in Circulating Blood Cells. A Sensitive Laboratory Test for the Detection of Childhood Lead Poisoning." *New England Journal of Medicine,* 284:565-569, 1971.

ENZYME INHIBITION BY LEAD
UNDER NORMAL URBAN CONDITIONS

S. HERNBERG   J. NIKKANEN

Summary A close negative correlation was found between the concentration of lead in blood and the activity of erythrocyte δ-aminolævulinic acid dehydrogenase in 26 healthy individuals, never exposed occupationally to lead. The results indicate that present levels of environmental contamination with lead can produce a measurable biochemical alteration in man.

INTRODUCTION

LEAD is absorbed into the human organism by respiratory and digestive routes and is distributed to organs and tissues by the bloodstream.[1] Metabolism is complex—some lead being excreted and some deposited; the rest forms a metabolically active pool reflected by the blood-level of lead.[1,2] As a result of growing industrial use and the introduction of alkyl lead compounds as petrol additives, exposure to lead is substantially above [3-9] the background of absorption from food and drinking-water. Epidemiological and experimental data point to a logarithmic correlation between the concentration of lead in the air and that in the blood of exposed individuals or populations,[7,8] suggesting that, in man, lead can accumulate as a result of increasing environmental contamination.

Any effect of the absorbed lead on health will depend on the degree of accumulation. The generally accepted " safe " upper limit for the concentration of lead in the blood of persons exposed industrially is some 70–80 μg. per 100 ml.,[1,2] and mean values for occupationally unexposed populations are usually between 15 and 25 μg. per 100 ml.[3,7,10] These levels are considered by most workers to be without any biological effects.

Inhibition of hæm synthesis is one manifestation of lead toxicity; and measurements of intermediate products of this metabolic chain—e.g., coproporphyrin and δ-aminolævulinic acid (A.L.A.) in urine—have long been used as quantitative tests of the response of the organism to surplus lead,[3,11] and have thus formed one basis for the evaluation of what is harmful and what is not. The finding that erythrocyte A.L.A. dehydrogenase activity is specifically inhibited by lead has provided a new, specific, and sensitive method for the detection of early lead effect.[11-13] We have used this test to see if measurable biological effects due to present levels of urban exposure to lead can be found in man.

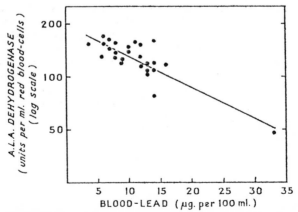

Relation between blood-lead and activity of erythrocyte A.L.A. dehydrogenase of 26 persons never occupationally exposed to lead.

B2

156

Blood-lead levels and erythrocyte A.L.A. dehydrogenase activity were measured in 26 healthy medical students (16 males, 10 females) with no present or previous occupational exposure to the metal. The concentration of lead in whole blood was measured after wet ashing using a dithizone method.[14] The standard deviation of duplicate measurements was $\pm 1 \cdot 3$ μg. per 100 ml. A blind control of the lead estimation gave the following result (the concentration in the blank sample recorded as 9 μg. per 100 ml.):

μg. per 100 ml.

Added	Measured
15	12
50	49
100	101

A.L.A. dehydrogenase was measured from fresh heparinised whole blood according to Bonsignore's method.[12] The results were corrected for hæmatocrit value, and the enzymatic activity was calculated from the formula:

$$1000 \times 12 \cdot 5 \ (A_{60} - A_0)/\text{hæmatocrit} \ (\%)$$

A_{60} and A_0 are the absorbencies at 60 and 0 minutes, respectively, and $12 \cdot 5$ is the dilution correction.

There was a strong negative correlation between the concentration of lead in the blood and the logarithm of A.L.A. dehydrogenase activity (see figure):

$$y = 2 \cdot 307 - 0 \cdot 018x; \ r = -0 \cdot 83$$

The results indicate that an inhibition of A.L.A. dehydrogenase that is proportional to the concentration of lead in the blood can be shown even for people representing " normal " urban exposure to lead. There is no lead level on the regression line below which it can be stated that no inhibition occurs.

We later extended our observations to 142 workers, representing various degrees of occupational exposure, with blood-lead values ranging from 11 to 94 μg. per 100 ml. The regression line was almost identical:

$$y = 2 \cdot 274 - 0 \cdot 018x; \ r = -0 \cdot 90$$

These observations confirm the results presented above and clearly show the interrelationship between the concentration of lead in the blood and the activity of A.L.A. dehydrogenase.

So far as we know, there have been no earlier reports indicating that present environmental contamination with lead has any biological effect on man. Our finding is an example of how the border between " effect " and " no effect " can be shifted by the introduction of more sensitive methods.

157

Indeed, inhibition of A.L.A. dehydrogenase was found at such low lead concentrations that one may ask whether there is any lead dose small enough to have no effect at all. The same may be true for other poisons; but a lack of sensitive methods for measuring toxic effects leaves this question open.

The effect of environmental contamination with lead on health has been subject to speculation.[1,4-6,15] The finding that A.L.A. dehydrogenase is partly inhibited in the " normal " urban population cannot be considered as proof of an effect on the health, since its significance is unknown as yet, but it demonstrates that even the comparatively low exposure to lead, prevailing today, interferes with metabolism. This interference may or may not be harmful. Without taking any standpoint on this question, it may be assumed from the Goldsmith-Hexter regression [8] that this and other possible effects will become more pronounced if contamination becomes heavier in the future.

We thank Miss Raili Vilhunen for her surveillance of the lead analyses.

Requests for reprints should be addressed to S. H.

REFERENCES

1. Kehoe, R. A. *Archs envir. Hlth*, 1964, **8**, 232.
2. Kehoe, R. A. *ibid*. p. 235.
3. Stopps, G. *J. occup. Med.* 1968, **10**, 550.
4. Patterson, C. C. *Archs envir. Hlth*, 1965, **11**, 344.
5. Schroeder, H. A., Tipton, I. H. *ibid*. 1968. **17**, 965.
6. Danielson, L. Report for the Swedish Royal Commission on Natural Resources. Solna, 1967.
7. *Publ. Hlth Ser. Publs, Wash.* 1965, no. 999-AP-12.
8. Goldsmith, J. R., Hexter, A. C. *Science*, 1967, **158**, 132.
9. Rühling, Å., Tyler, G. *Bot. Notiser*, 1968, **121**, 21.
10. Hofreuter, D. H., Catcott, E. J., Keenan, R. G., Xintaras, G. *Archs envir. Hlth*, 1961, **3**, 568.
11. De Bruin, A. *Med. Lavoro*, 1968, **59**, 411.
12. Bonsignore, D. *ibid*. 1966, **57**, 647.
13. Nakao, K., Wada, O., Yano, Y. *Clin. Chimica Acta*, 1968, **19**, 319.
14. Keenan, R. G., Byers, D. H., Salzman, B. E., Hyslop, F. L. *Am. ind. Hyg. Ass.* 1963, **24**, 481.
15. Haley, T. J. *Archs envir. Hlth*, 1966, **12**, 781.

158

Occupational Exposure To Toxic Levels Of Lead

BODY BURDEN, DISTRIBUTION AND INTERNAL DOSE OF ^{210}PB AND ^{210}PO IN A URANIUM MINER POPULATION

R. L. BLANCHARD and J. B. MOORE

INTRODUCTION

MUCH HIGHER than normal concentrations of ^{210}Po and ^{210}Pb have been observed in the skeletons of uranium miners.[1-3] The sources of ^{210}Pb which contribute to these high skeletal burdens are: (1) inhalation of short-lived radon daughters with subsequent decay in the lung to ^{210}Pb, of which a fraction is absorbed into the blood stream and stored in the skeleton,[1,2] (2) inhalation and possibly ingestion of ^{210}Pb present in the mine atmosphere,[2,4] and (3) inhalation of ^{222}Rn which is stored in body fat; upon decay, the daughters translocate via the blood stream to the skeleton.[5] The first two sources contribute by far the largest fraction of the ^{210}Pb to the body burden. It has been estimated that ^{222}Rn inhalation will normally contribute less than 10%.[2,5] Since the ^{210}Po/^{210}Pb activity ratio is small in mine air, generally less than 10%,[4] most ^{210}Po present in the body of a miner is due to the decay of stored ^{210}Pb.

The purpose of this investigation was to obtain information on the body burden and distribution within the body of ^{210}Pb and ^{210}Po, to calculate the radiation dose delivered by ^{210}Po to the more critical body compartments, and to investigate further the relationship which has been reported to exist between the concentration of ^{210}Pb in blood to that in the skeleton.[2] The high concentrations present in the tissues of uranium miners make it possible to investigate tissues and portions of organs which in non-exposed individuals are too low to measure accurately. Hopefully, information obtained here may be related to population groups other than uranium miners.

The concentration of ^{210}Pb has been reported in bone samples from more than 50 miners, but ^{210}Po concentrations were obtained in less than half of these samples. Also, little data have been reported on the ^{210}Pb and ^{210}Po soft tissue concentrations of this exposed population. As certain soft tissues have been shown to concentrate ^{210}Po,[6,7] one of the more hazardous radioactive elements,[8] the dose delivered to some tissues by ^{210}Po may be significant.

METHODS

Samples of whole rib, vertebra, organ and tissue were obtained from the subjects at autopsy or surgery. Each tissue, including bone, was cut into 2 mm slices and pathologically examined. Abnormal or diseased tissue was removed and either analyzed separately or discarded.

Measured quantities of blood, about 20 ml, were taken at autopsy. Although it would have been preferable to have obtained the blood sample prior to the subject's death, it was not feasible.

Du   he thermal volatility of ^{210}Po, the bone ....p..cs could not be dry ashed. The bone samples were defatted in anhydrous benzene in order to give a reproducible bone sample weight,[9] and it was determined that neither ^{210}Po nor ^{210}Pb were removed during the extraction. The average ratio of defat weight/fresh weight was 0.46 ± 0.07 (S.D.) for rib and 0.33 ± 0.04 (S.D.) for vertebra.

The analytical procedure employed to determine ^{210}Po and ^{210}Pb has been described previously.[7,10] The samples were wet ashed in nitric acid and 72% perchloric acid and the ^{210}Po was deposited on a 2 in. silver disc from a 0.5 N HCl solution containing 200 mg of ascorbic acid at 85°C. The ^{210}Pb present was calculated from the ^{210}Po ingrowth which was measured by repeating the ^{210}Po deposition on another silver disc 3–4 months after the initial deposition. The alpha activity of the ^{210}Po deposited on the disc was measured in a low-background (0.2–0.8 counts/hr) ZnS(Ag) scintillation counter. The ^{210}Po values were corrected for decay and ingrowth from ^{210}Pb to obtain the concentration at the time of the miners' death or surgery.

RESULTS

The 54 men whose tissues were studied are listed in the order of increasing exposure in Table 1. The age of the miners at death or surgery varied from 28 to 73 yr. All cases listed died with lung cancer except 04, 17 and 23 whose deaths were attributed to bronchopneumonia with severe pulmonary emphysema, and 12 and 13 whose samples were obtained at surgery. Eleven of the cases were non-miners who had resided in the Colorado Plateau region. The column listing years of hardrock mining refers to other than uranium mining. Since cigarette smoking has been shown to elevate the ^{210}Po concentration in some tissues, smoking data have been listed in the last two columns.[6,11–14]

The exposures listed in Table 1 are given in units of "working-level-months" (WLM), which are based upon atmospheric measurements made in the uranium mines.[15] The working-level factor (WL) has been described in detail.[16] Briefly, the working level (WL) is a unit of the concentration of radon daughters in air, and is defined as any combination of radon daughters

162

per liter of air which will result in the emission of 1.3×10^5 MeV of alpha energy upon complete decay to ^{210}Pb. The working level month (WLM) is a unit of exposure to radon daughters in air, and is defined as an exposure to a concentration of one working level for a duration equivalent to 170 hr. The duration of exposure in months was obtained by interviewing the miner and/or his surviving relatives. In addition to exposure in uranium mines, an exposure of 1 WL has been assigned for other hardrock mining prior to 1935, 0.5 WL for 1935–1940 and 0.3 WL for other hardrock mining exposures after 1940.[15] Factors which place a degree of uncertainty on these exposure values are the variation in radon-daughter concentrations in mine air with time and ventilation, the movement of miners from one location to another in a mine, the particle size distribution of mine dust on which the radon daughters collect, the variations in physiological parameters among individuals, the mine sampling data which necessitated the use of estimates for some of the mining exposures, and the recall accuracy of the individuals interviewed.

Listed in Table 2 are the concentrations of ^{210}Po and ^{210}Pb measured in the various tissues, and in the last column are given the ^{210}Po/^{210}Pb activity ratios. The uncertainties listed are for a one standard deviation counting error. Generally, concentrations observed in healthy tissue are listed. In some cases, however, the tissue was so infested by tumors that sufficient healthy tissue was not available. The occurrence of the latter is noted in Table 2 by an asterisk.

The results shown in Table 3 are representative of those which have previously been reported for tissue taken from individuals with no record of exposure to either ^{210}Po or ^{210}Pb. The average values are given along with the range in parenthesis. The results are given on the basis of fresh weights for soft tissues and ash weights for bone. The asterisks indicate cigarette smokers. These values will be used as a basis for comparison with the tissue samples of this study.

The analytical data listed in Table 2 will

Table 1. *Exposure data of uranium miners and non-mining adult males sampled*

Miner No.	Age	Exposure (WLM)	End of mining to death (yrs)	Uranium mining (yrs)	Hard rock mining (yrs)*	Cigarettes per day	Years of smoking
01	67	0	—	0	0	20	35
02	57	0	—	0	0	30	40
03	69	0	—	0	0	3	61
04	71	0	—	0	0	40	40
05	63	0	—	0	0	20	53
06	58	0	—	0	0	30	15
07	59	0	—	0	0	20	41
08	59	0	—	0	0	30	32
09	54	0	—	0	0	40	38
10	50	0	—	0	0	20	37
11	66	0	—	0	0	4 and pipe	10
12	28	80	$6\frac{1}{4}$	$\frac{1}{3}$	0	NA	NA
13	34	102	2	5	0	15	19
14	60	126	$\frac{1}{12}$	0	30	20	30
15	53	138	$\frac{1}{2}$	$5\frac{3}{8}$	0	25	20
16	67	150	43	0	1	40	54
17	72	180	20	0	37	20	55
18	41	183	$7\frac{1}{4}$	$1\frac{1}{2}$	0	30	25
19	49	208	1	$\frac{1}{2}$	5	20	30
20	46	242	$\frac{3}{4}$	6	13	30	29
21	60	320	10	$2\frac{2}{3}$	27	25	35
22	51	408	$\frac{5}{6}$	8	2	20	24
23	57	435	9	$2\frac{1}{2}$	0	18	39
24	53	544	$3\frac{1}{2}$	$5\frac{1}{2}$	15	10	29
25	45	548	8	$\frac{3}{4}$	2	12	31
26	46	604	11	$2\frac{1}{2}$	12	20	27
27	50	727	$2\frac{1}{6}$	$10\frac{1}{4}$	5	20	38
28	62	743	1	$8\frac{1}{2}$	20	30 and pipe	33
29	59	826	2	14	7	30	35
30	60	845	$1\frac{1}{3}$	9	13	5	35
31	56	1070	$\frac{1}{6}$	$5\frac{1}{2}$	25	25	10
32	57	1083	$1\frac{1}{2}$	11	$1\frac{1}{2}$	20	27
33	65	1098	1	12	0	15	51
34	56	1161	$\frac{1}{12}$	11	0	0	0
35	52	1293	$\frac{1}{12}$	19	9	20	37
36	49	1385	$\frac{3}{4}$	$7\frac{1}{2}$	19	20	38
37	61	1400	25	6	0	20	40
38	55	1444	$\frac{1}{12}$	8	13	20	40
39	73	1490	18	30	5	0	0
40	55	1846	$6\frac{1}{2}$	6	0	0	0
41	50	1880	$\frac{1}{12}$	15	17	4 cigars	25
42	58	1951	$\frac{1}{2}$	20	0	35	40
43	64	2173	7	11	7	30	25
44	73	2342	11	8	0	15	45
45	50	2506	$\frac{1}{4}$	15	0	20	35
46	44	2635	$\frac{1}{3}$	$13\frac{1}{2}$	4	20	20
47	55	2818	$4\frac{1}{4}$	14	4	20	37
48	46	2885	$\frac{1}{2}$	15	0	20	27
49	59	2890	6	$10\frac{1}{2}$	4	20	25
50	61	3000	35	5	0	15	35
51	56	3220	$1\frac{1}{2}$	20	0	15	NA
52	55	3588	3	10	10	30	37
53	60	4357	$\frac{1}{6}$	27	0	20	45
54	50	4373	$2\frac{1}{2}$	14	20	20	40

* Other than uranium mining.
NA—information not available.

Table 2. Concentrations of ^{210}Po and ^{210}Pb in uranium miner tissues

Miner No.	^{210}Po (pCi/kg)	^{210}Pb (pCi/kg)	^{210}Po/^{210}Pb	Miner No.	^{210}Po (pCi/kg)	^{210}Pb (pCi/kg)	^{210}Po/^{210}Pb
	Lung and associated tissues			26-P	184 ± 8	250 ± 10	0.74 ± 0.05
				26-L	302 ± 12	576 ± 44	0.53 ± 0.05
01	—	12 ± 2	—	26-B	37 ± 5	96 ± 16	0.39 ± 0.08
02*	—	5.4 ± 0.5	—	27	282 ± 4	565 ± 9	0.50 ± 0.01
03	—	12 ± 1	—	27-P	356 ± 5	590 ± 11	0.61 ± 0.01
03-L	—	45 ± 6	—	27-L	504 ± 40	695 ± 70	0.73 ± 0.09
04	—	12.3 ± 0.6	—	28	—	161 ± 2	—
04-P	—	17.9 ± 0.8	—	28-P	—	182 ± 4	—
04-L	—	38 ± 3	—	28-L	—	211 ± 21	—
05	7.4 ± 0.4	9.8 ± 0.9	0.75 ± 0.08	29	353 ± 4	406 ± 6	0.86 ± 0.02
05-P	8.6 ± 0.7	15 ± 1	0.59 ± 0.07	29-P	438 ± 6	460 ± 10	0.95 ± 0.03
06	6.0 ± 0.4	9.2 ± 0.8	0.65 ± 0.07	29-L	1380 ± 30	1730 ± 50	0.80 ± 0.03
06-P	6.9 ± 0.5	9.5 ± 0.8	0.73 ± 0.08	30	—	379 ± 6	—
06-L	17 ± 2	20 ± 4	0.85 ± 0.20	30-P*	—	210 ± 6	—
07*	—	7.4 ± 0.4	—	30-L*	—	27 ± 3	—
07-P	—	15 ± 1	—	31	12.2 ± 0.5	26 ± 1	0.47 ± 0.03
08*	—	6.6 ± 0.6	—	31-P	29 ± 1	32 ± 2	0.91 ± 0.07
08-P*	—	16 ± 1	—	31-L	344 ± 8	414 ± 14	0.83 ± 0.03
09	—	8.0 ± 0.6	—	32	—	1300 ± 16	—
10*	—	8.6 ± 0.6	—	33	1120 ± 6	1850 ± 13	0.61 ± 0.01
10-P*	—	11 ± 1	—	33-P	1350 ± 14	1760 ± 18	0.77 ± 0.01
11	5.0 ± 0.3	6.1 ± 0.6	0.81 ± 0.10	35	467 ± 4	930 ± 10	0.50 ± 0.01
11-P	8.5 ± 0.6	12 ± 1	0.74 ± 0.08	35-P	710 ± 7	1120 ± 12	0.63 ± 0.01
11-L	37 ± 4	48 ± 6	0.77 ± 0.12	35-L	900 ± 12	1270 ± 20	0.71 ± 0.02
13	—	74 ± 3	—	36	—	482 ± 8	—
13-P	—	97 ± 8	—	37*	—	29 ± 1	—
14	3.7 ± 0.2	7.0 ± 0.7	0.53 ± 0.06	37-P*	—	42 ± 1	—
14-P	4.7 ± 0.4	8.3 ± 0.8	0.57 ± 0.07	37-L*	—	177 ± 6	—
15*	—	340 ± 4	—	38	1380 ± 10	2500 ± 25	0.55 ± 0.01
16	—	9.3 ± 0.9	—	38-P	2650 ± 30	2980 ± 40	0.89 ± 0.01
16-P*	—	23 ± 2	—	38-L*	606 ± 10	1010 ± 23	0.60 ± 0.02
17	3.6 ± 0.2	4.5 ± 0.4	0.80 ± 0.09	40	547 ± 7	765 ± 12	0.72 ± 0.02
17-P	9.8 ± 0.5	15 ± 1	0.65 ± 0.05	40-P	643 ± 7	797 ± 14	0.81 ± 0.02
17-L	17 ± 3	41 ± 5	0.43 ± 0.08	40-L	1710 ± 30	1710 ± 40	1.00 ± 0.03
18	—	73 ± 2	—	41	229 ± 3	244 ± 5	0.94 ± 0.02
19	—	132 ± 4	—	41-P*	269 ± 5	282 ± 8	0.95 ± 0.03
19-P	—	242 ± 7	—	41-L*	57 ± 4	83 ± 8	0.69 ± 0.08
19-L	—	614 ± 32	—	42	—	342 ± 5	—
20	165 ± 7	346 ± 20	0.48 ± 0.04	42-P	—	435 ± 8	—
20-L	455 ± 4	594 ± 8	0.77 ± 0.01	43	—	260 ± 4	—
21	—	187 ± 5	—	43-P*	—	293 ± 6	—
21-P	—	217 ± 5	—	43-L*	—	889 ± 15	—
21-L	—	316 ± 9	—	44	54 ± 2	59 ± 3	0.92 ± 0.06
22	—	225 ± 5	—	44-P	95 ± 4	148 ± 9	0.64 ± 0.05
22-P	—	520 ± 10	—	44-L	156 ± 6	228 ± 18	0.68 ± 0.06
23	—	206 ± 3	—	45	1040 ± 12	1380 ± 23	0.75 ± 0.02
23-P	—	205 ± 2	—	46	156 ± 4	198 ± 6	0.78 ± 0.03
23-L	—	515 ± 15	—	46-P	258 ± 5	323 ± 9	0.80 ± 0.03
24	—	91 ± 3	—	47	520 ± 4	708 ± 16	0.73 ± 0.02
25	—	97 ± 4	—	47-P	764 ± 5	1030 ± 16	0.74 ± 0.01
26	142 ± 3	140 ± 5	1.00 ± 0.04	48	1200 ± 14	1580 ± 20	0.75 ± 0.02

165

Table 2.—(contd.)

Miner No.	^{210}Po (pCi/kg)	^{210}Pb (pCi/kg)	^{210}Po/^{210}Pb
Lung and associated tissues			
48-P	1800 ± 10	2310 ± 30	0.78 ± 0.01
49*	686 ± 6	933 ± 11	0.74 ± 0.01
50	19.0 ± 0.7	25 ± 1	0.76 ± 0.05
50-P	29 ± 1	45 ± 3	0.65 ± 0.05
50-L*	61 ± 5	266 ± 17	0.23 ± 0.02
51	—	142 ± 5	—
51-L	—	677 ± 36	—
52	322 ± 4	377 ± 5	0.99 ± 0.02
52-L	511 ± 13	578 ± 20	0.88 ± 0.04
52-B	34 ± 3	70 ± 7	0.49 ± 0.06
53	—	174 ± 4	—
53-P	—	295 ± 10	—
53-L	—	990 ± 70	—
54*	—	329 ± 5	—
Liver			
02	5.5 ± 0.3	10.0 ± 0.7	0.55 ± 0.05
11	16.1 ± 0.8	9.6 ± 0.9	1.7 ± 0.2
13	55 ± 2	32 ± 2	1.7 ± 0.1
18	62 ± 1	31 ± 2	2.0 ± 0.1
20	88 ± 2	25 ± 1	3.5 ± 0.2
22	61 ± 1	87 ± 3	0.70 ± 0.03
23	14.7 ± 0.6	22 ± 1	0.67 ± 0.05
24	24.0 ± 0.8	35 ± 2	0.68 ± 0.04
25	126 ± 1	175 ± 4	0.72 ± 0.02
26	157 ± 2	118 ± 3	1.33 ± 0.04
27	96 ± 2	26 ± 2	3.7 ± 0.3
28	86 ± 2	126 ± 3	0.68 ± 0.02
29	—	124 ± 2	—
33	276 ± 8	208 ± 12	1.33 ± 0.08
36	183 ± 2	184 ± 4	1.02 ± 0.03
37	—	48 ± 1	—
38*	87 ± 1	91 ± 2	0.96 ± 0.03
40	76 ± 1	75 ± 2	1.01 ± 0.03
41*	75 ± 2	51 ± 2	1.45 ± 0.06
43	307 ± 3	404 ± 3	0.76 ± 0.01
44*	35.0 ± 0.6	25 ± 1	1.38 ± 0.07
45	480 ± 8	399 ± 11	1.20 ± 0.04
47	305 ± 2	410 ± 7	0.75 ± 0.02
48	685 ± 6	830 ± 10	0.83 ± 0.02
50	—	135 ± 3	—
51*	95 ± 2	120 ± 3	0.79 ± 0.03
52*	150 ± 3	222 ± 4	0.68 ± 0.02
53	234 ± 3	201 ± 4	1.16 ± 0.03
Kidney (cortex)			
02	14 ± 1	6.4 ± 0.6	2.2 ± 0.2
11	19 ± 1	4.7 ± 0.6	4.0 ± 0.6
13	78 ± 3	16 ± 1	4.9 ± 0.5

Miner No.	^{210}Po (pCi/kg)	^{210}Pb (pCi/kg)	^{210}Po/^{210}Pb
18	190 ± 3	17.4 ± 0.7	10.9 ± 0.5
20	131 ± 3	21 ± 2	6.2 ± 0.7
22	143 ± 2	25 ± 1	5.7 ± 0.3
23	32 ± 1	11 ± 1	3.0 ± 0.3
24	77 ± 1	11 ± 1	7.0 ± 0.8
25	210 ± 3	36 ± 2	5.8 ± 0.3
26	145 ± 2	22 ± 1	6.6 ± 0.4
27	377 ± 7	120 ± 5	3.1 ± 0.2
28	295 ± 4	16 ± 1	18 ± 1
29	—	57 ± 2	—
33	693 ± 6	75 ± 3	9.2 ± 0.4
36	268 ± 3	89 ± 3	3.0 ± 0.1
37	—	50 ± 3	—
38	726 ± 8	88 ± 3	8.2 ± 0.3
40	49 ± 2	26 ± 2	1.9 ± 0.2
41	164 ± 3	26 ± 1	6.4 ± 0.4
43	258 ± 4	61 ± 1	4.2 ± 0.1
44	40 ± 1	12 ± 1	3.3 ± 0.4
47	728 ± 4	78 ± 3	9.3 ± 0.4
48	1498 ± 13	70 ± 3	21 ± 1
50	—	33 ± 1	—
51	314 ± 5	14.4 ± 0.9	22 ± 2
52	181 ± 3	12 ± 1	16 ± 1
53	921 ± 11	36 ± 2	25 ± 2
Spleen			
02	1.3 ± 0.4	1.7 ± 0.4	0.76 ± 0.21
18	16.0 ± 0.5	40 ± 2	0.41 ± 0.02
20	14.1 ± 0.6	38 ± 2	0.37 ± 0.02
22	11 ± 1	26 ± 2	0.42 ± 0.05
23	14.0 ± 0.6	46 ± 2	0.30 ± 0.02
24	5.7 ± 0.4	11.2 ± 0.9	0.51 ± 0.05
25	26 ± 1	100 ± 3	0.26 ± 0.01
27	2.6 ± 0.2	4.8 ± 0.5	0.53 ± 0.07
33	54 ± 1	225 ± 5	0.24 ± 0.01
36	16.3 ± 0.5	44 ± 2	0.37 ± 0.02
38	53 ± 1	192 ± 4	0.28 ± 0.01
40	45 ± 2	54 ± 2	0.83 ± 0.05
41	24 ± 1	28 ± 2	0.86 ± 0.06
43	61 ± 1	97 ± 2	0.63 ± 0.01
44	8.3 ± 0.4	11.4 ± 0.8	0.73 ± 0.06
47	73 ± 2	150 ± 4	0.49 ± 0.02
48	167 ± 6	160 ± 9	1.04 ± 0.07
51	35 ± 1	68 ± 3	0.51 ± 0.03
52	23.1 ± 0.7	90 ± 3	0.26 ± 0.01
53	31 ± 1	128 ± 2	0.24 ± 0.01
Testes			
02	2.5 ± 0.1	1.2 ± 0.2	2.1 ± 0.2
11	4.8 ± 0.5	2.2 ± 0.4	2.2 ± 0.5

Table 2.—(contd.)

Testes

Miner No.	^{210}Po (pCi/kg)	^{210}Pb (pCi/kg)	^{210}Po/^{210}Pb
13	15.4 ± 0.9	4.4 ± 0.7	3.5 ± 0.6
18	23 ± 2	4.0 ± 0.6	6 ± 1
20	29 ± 2	7.8 ± 1.0	3.7 ± 0.5
22	34 ± 2	9 ± 1	3.8 ± 0.5
23	7.0 ± 0.6	5.1 ± 0.7	1.4 ± 0.2
24	14 ± 1	4.6 ± 0.7	3.0 ± 0.5
25	31 ± 2	3.3 ± 0.5	9.4 ± 0.6
26	41 ± 2	4.3 ± 0.5	10 ± 1
27	28 ± 1	7.0 ± 0.4	4.0 ± 0.3
28	35 ± 2	9 ± 1	3.9 ± 0.5
29	—	20 ± 1	—
33	149 ± 4	20 ± 2	7.4 ± 0.8
36	66 ± 4	26 ± 1	2.5 ± 0.2
37	—	11.2 ± 0.9	—
38	54 ± 2	19 ± 1	2.8 ± 0.2
40	19 ± 1	5.5 ± 0.7	3.7 ± 0.6
41	30 ± 1	5.3 ± 0.7	5.7 ± 0.8
43	106 ± 4	29 ± 2	3.7 ± 0.3
47	95 ± 3	11 ± 1	8.6 ± 0.8
48	149 ± 3	18 ± 2	8.3 ± 0.8
50	—	26 ± 1	—
51	117 ± 5	32 ± 2	3.7 ± 0.3
52	43 ± 2	6.3 ± 0.8	7 ± 1

Heart

Miner No.	^{210}Po (pCi/kg)	^{210}Pb (pCi/kg)	^{210}Po/^{210}Pb
02	2.4 ± 0.2	4.1 ± 0.6	0.59 ± 0.09
18	11.7 ± 0.7	6.2 ± 0.6	1.9 ± 0.2
20	5.3 ± 0.4	4.7 ± 0.6	1.1 ± 0.1
22	5.7 ± 0.4	13 ± 1	0.38 ± 0.05
23	1.4 ± 0.2	2.5 ± 0.4	0.6 ± 0.1
24	2.7 ± 0.1	3.4 ± 0.5	0.8 ± 0.1
25	11.0 ± 0.8	6.0 ± 0.5	1.8 ± 0.2
26	7.5 ± 0.5	3.5 ± 0.4	2.1 ± 0.3
27	4.2 ± 0.3	2.3 ± 0.3	1.8 ± 0.3
29	—	8.1 ± 0.5	—
30	6.0 ± 0.4	4.8 ± 0.6	1.3 ± 0.2
33	26 ± 1	18 ± 1	1.4 ± 0.1
36	12.7 ± 0.5	9.9 ± 0.6	1.3 ± 0.1
38	12.0 ± 0.6	15 ± 1	0.82 ± 0.08
40	9.0 ± 0.3	4.9 ± 0.3	1.8 ± 0.2
41	9.4 ± 0.5	15 ± 1	0.62 ± 0.06
43	15.7 ± 0.6	11.1 ± 0.5	1.4 ± 0.1
44	2.5 ± 0.1	3.6 ± 0.5	0.7 ± 0.1
47	12.7 ± 0.7	16 ± 1	0.79 ± 0.07
48	26 ± 1	21 ± 2	1.2 ± 0.1
50	—	7.3 ± 0.4	—
51	6.0 ± 0.4	8.6 ± 0.6	0.70 ± 0.07
53	24.8 ± 0.8	13.0 ± 0.8	1.90 ± 0.1
54	9.0 ± 0.3	7.0 ± 0.6	1.3 ± 0.1

Muscle

Miner No.	^{210}Po (pCi/kg)	^{210}Pb (pCi/kg)	^{210}Po/^{210}Pb
02	2.2 ± 0.2	2.9 ± 0.4	0.8 ± 0.2
11	1.7 ± 0.3	1.2 ± 0.3	1.4 ± 0.4
13	3.8 ± 0.3	9.5 ± 0.8	0.40 ± 0.05
18	4.6 ± 0.3	3.0 ± 0.3	1.5 ± 0.2
20	7.6 ± 0.4	11.6 ± 0.6	0.66 ± 0.06
23	1.1 ± 0.2	2.1 ± 0.4	0.5 ± 0.1
24	2.7 ± 0.3	2.4 ± 0.4	1.1 ± 0.2
26	2.6 ± 0.3	2.7 ± 0.4	1.0 ± 0.2
27	3.6 ± 0.3	7.0 ± 0.6	0.52 ± 0.06
28	9.9 ± 0.7	6.0 ± 0.7	1.6 ± 0.2
22	4.7 ± 0.3	11.3 ± 0.9	0.42 ± 0.04
33	16 ± 1	17 ± 1	0.94 ± 0.05
36	8.2 ± 0.4	6.0 ± 0.5	1.4 ± 0.1
38	8.4 ± 0.4	4.9 ± 0.5	1.7 ± 0.2
40	7.2 ± 0.4	6.2 ± 0.6	1.2 ± 0.1
41	5.5 ± 0.4	11 ± 1	0.50 ± 0.06
43	8.2 ± 0.5	9.3 ± 0.5	0.88 ± 0.07
29	—	3.2 ± 0.3	—
44	6.5 ± 0.7	5.1 ± 0.5	1.3 ± 0.2
47	11.5 ± 0.6	7.2 ± 0.8	1.6 ± 0.2
48	36 ± 2	32 ± 2	1.1 ± 0.1
51	14.4 ± 0.6	8.5 ± 0.5	1.7 ± 0.1
52	2.2 ± 0.2	3.0 ± 0.3	0.7 ± 0.1
53	17.2 ± 0.7	6.6 ± 0.5	2.6 ± 0.2

Lymph nodes

Miner No.	^{210}Po (pCi/kg)	^{210}Pb (pCi/kg)	^{210}Po/^{210}Pb
11	21 ± 2	30 ± 3	0.7 ± 0.1
13*	19 ± 2	28 ± 3	0.7 ± 0.1
18	56 ± 2	83 ± 4	0.68 ± 0.04
20	188 ± 4	278 ± 9	0.68 ± 0.03
24	143 ± 3	133 ± 8	1.08 ± 0.06
26	57 ± 4	63 ± 6	0.9 ± 0.1
28	274 ± 8	350 ± 16	0.78 ± 0.04
30	—	178 ± 19	—
33	100 ± 8	82 ± 7	1.2 ± 0.2
44*	21 ± 2	36 ± 4	0.59 ± 0.09
47	1300 ± 60	1740 ± 70	0.75 ± 0.04
48*	83 ± 12	280 ± 40	0.30 ± 0.07
50*	—	10 ± 1	—
54	340 ± 6	410 ± 10	0.83 ± 0.03

Pancreas

Miner No.	^{210}Po (pCi/kg)	^{210}Pb (pCi/kg)	^{210}Po/^{210}Pb
18	17 ± 1	15 ± 1	1.1 ± 0.1
25	21 ± 1	20 ± 2	1.1 ± 0.1
33	71 ± 2	22 ± 2	3.2 ± 0.3
36	15.6 ± 0.7	17 ± 1	0.93 ± 0.07
38	22 ± 1	39 ± 3	0.56 ± 0.05
44	4.0 ± 0.2	3.7 ± 0.4	1.1 ± 0.1
48	97 ± 2	53 ± 3~	1.8 ± 0.1
53	44 ± 3	22 ± 2	2.0 ± 0.2

Table 2.—(contd.)

Miner No.	^{210}Po (pCi/kg)	^{210}Pb (pCi/kg)	^{210}Po/^{210}Pb	Miner No.	^{210}Po (pCi/kg)	^{210}Pb (pCi/kg)	^{210}Po/^{210}Pb
	Aorta			28-V*	1310 ± 20	1960 ± 50	0.67 ± 0.02
22	5 ± 1	14 ± 3	0.4 ± 0.1	29-R	2720 ± 40	3800 ± 40	0.72 ± 0.01
28	284 ± 6	330 ± 10	0.86 ± 0.03	31-R	1760 ± 20	2160 ± 40	0.81 ± 0.03
28a	690 ± 11	1160 ± 26	0.60 ± 0.02	33-R	2750 ± 20	5010 ± 60	0.55 ± 0.01
38	220 ± 4	324 ± 10	0.68 ± 0.02	33-V	3250 ± 30	5220 ± 70	0.63 ± 0.01
54	508 ± 12	588 ± 16	0.86 ± 0.03	34-R	1440 ± 20	2500 ± 40	0.58 ± 0.01
54a	678 ± 11	787 ± 25	0.86 ± 0.03	36-R	3950 ± 40	4260 ± 60	0.93 ± 0.02
				36-V	3240 ± 40	4600 ± 60	0.70 ± 0.01
	Adrenal gland			37-R	910 ± 6	813 ± 10	1.12 ± 0.02
22*	17 ± 2	33 ± 4	0.52 ± 0.08	38-R	4180 ± 40	7180 ± 80	0.58 ± 0.01
25	49 ± 4	14 ± 2	3.4 ± 0.5	39-R	1050 ± 20	1150 ± 30	0.91 ± 0.03
36	80 ± 4	18 ± 2	4.4 ± 0.5	40-R	1320 ± 20	1760 ± 40	0.75 ± 0.03
48	217 ± 6	46 ± 5	2.8 ± 0.3	40-V	1690 ± 20	1900 ± 40	0.89 ± 0.02
				41-R	2070 ± 30	1740 ± 40	1.19 ± 0.04
	Prostate			41-V	1680 ± 20	2240 ± 50	0.75 ± 0.02
36	23 ± 2	20 ± 2	1.2 ± 0.2	43-R	1750 ± 20	2720 ± 50	0.64 ± 0.01
53	21 ± 3	42 ± 5	0.50 ± 0.09	43-V	1870 ± 20	2530 ± 50	0.74 ± 0.02
				44-R	1310 ± 20	1390 ± 30	0.94 ± 0.03
	Thyroid			44-V	1180 ± 20	1400 ± 30	0.84 ± 0.02
48	90 ± 4	60 ± 6	1.5 ± 0.2	45-R	1570 ± 20	1690 ± 40	0.93 ± 0.03
				47-R	4010 ± 30	5030 ± 60	0.80 ± 0.01
	Bone			47-V	5660 ± 50	6640 ± 70	0.85 ± 0.01
02-R	93 ± 6	98 ± 8	0.95 ± 0.10	48-R	4890 ± 30	5730 ± 50	0.85 ± 0.01
02-V	85 ± 6	90 ± 8	0.94 ± 0.10	48-V	5860 ± 40	9580 ± 90	0.62 ± 0.01
11-R	90 ± 6	135 ± 12	0.67 ± 0.08	48-S	2740 ± 40	3450 ± 50	0.79 ± 0.02
11-V	75 ± 6	140 ± 14	0.54 ± 0.07	49-R	4110 ± 20	4630 ± 50	0.89 ± 0.01
12-R	405 ± 10	529 ± 20	0.77 ± 0.03	50-R	1600 ± 20	1800 ± 30	0.89 ± 0.02
13-R	209 ± 4	360 ± 10	0.82 ± 0.04	51-R	4250 ± 40	5110 ± 50	0.83 ± 0.01
13-V	428 ± 11	677 ± 25	0.63 ± 0.03	51-V	3920 ± 40	4200 ± 50	0.94 ± 0.02
18-R	549 ± 14	937 ± 26	0.59 ± 0.02	52-R	3150 ± 40	4360 ± 60	0.72 ± 0.01
18-V	500 ± 15	768 ± 24	0.65 ± 0.03	52-V	2570 ± 30	3000 ± 40	0.86 ± 0.02
20-R	1780 ± 25	2870 ± 50	0.62 ± 0.01	53-R	2240 ± 20	5830 ± 60	0.39 ± 0.01
20-V	1040 ± 18	1530 ± 30	0.68 ± 0.02	53-V	3460 ± 30	4310 ± 50	0.80 ± 0.01
22-R	650 ± 10	1380 ± 30	0.47 ± 0.01				
22-V	760 ± 18	1500 ± 45	0.51 ± 0.02		Spinal cord		
22-S	520 ± 12	850 ± 30	0.61 ± 0.03	18	5 ± 1	7 ± 1	0.7 ± 0.2
23-R	198 ± 7	292 ± 13	0.68 ± 0.04	20	11 ± 1	16 ± 2	0.7 ± 0.1
23-V*	162 ± 6	210 ± 13	0.77 ± 0.04	26	12 ± 2	14 ± 2	0.9 ± 0.2
23-S*	183 ± 7	234 ± 12	0.78 ± 0.05	38	8 ± 1	32 ± 2	0.25 ± 0.03
24-R	415 ± 12	408 ± 17	1.02 ± 0.05	48	33 ± 2	160 ± 16	0.21 ± 0.03
24-V	453 ± 14	630 ± 24	0.72 ± 0.03	51	11 ± 1	12 ± 2	0.9 ± 0.2
25-R	1830 ± 25	3060 ± 45	0.61 ± 0.01	53	24 ± 3	30 ± 4	0.8 ± 0.1
25-V	1800 ± 29	2650 ± 44	0.68 ± 0.02				
26-R	1550 ± 20	1880 ± 30	0.83 ± 0.02		Small intestine		
26-V	1485 ± 20	1710 ± 30	0.87 ± 0.02	18	13 ± 1	5.6 ± 0.5	2.4 ± 0.3
27-R	1280 ± 20	2260 ± 40	0.57 ± 0.01	25	13.2 ± 0.8	6.0 ± 0.5	2.2 ± 0.2
28-R	1200 ± 20	1330 ± 30	0.90 ± 0.03	36	33 ± 1	18 ± 1	1.8 ± 0.2
				40	13.6 ± 0.7	8.6 ± 0.8	1.6 ± 0.2

Table 2.—(contd.)

Miner No.	^{210}Po (pCi/kg)	^{210}Pb (pCi/kg)	^{210}Po/^{210}Pb
Small intestine			
48	393 ± 12	180 ± 16	2.2 ± 0.2
52	24 ± 1	9.0 ± 0.8	2.7 ± 0.3
53	41 ± 1	18 ± 1	2.2 ± 0.2
Brain			
52a	14 ± 1	8 ± 1	1.8 ± 0.3
52b	13.5 ± 0.8	8.5 ± 0.7	1.6 ± 0.2
Stomach			
18	10.6 ± 0.9	4.1 ± 0.5	2.6 ± 0.4
36	20 ± 1	16 ± 1	1.3 ± 0.1
53	33 ± 2	20 ± 2	1.7 ± 0.2
Blood			
11	0.40 ± 0.08	1.8 ± 0.3	0.24 ± 0.05
12	5.3 ± 0.6	15 ± 2	0.36 ± 0.06

Miner No.	^{210}Po (pCi/kg)	^{210}Pb (pCi/kg)	^{210}Po/^{210}Pb
13	4.8 ± 0.2	6.6 ± 0.8	0.73 ± 0.05
18	5.0 ± 0.4	10 ± 1	0.50 ± 0.08
22	7.0 ± 0.5	27 ± 2	0.26 ± 0.03
24	3.0 ± 0.2	9 ± 1	0.33 ± 0.04
26	16 ± 1	33 ± 2	0.47 ± 0.05
29	8.2 ± 0.5	27 ± 1	0.30 ± 0.03
33	15 ± 1	38 ± 2	0.40 ± 0.06
36	11.4 ± 0.8	48 ± 4	0.24 ± 0.03
37	—	11 ± 1	—
38	35 ± 1	122 ± 3	0.29 ± 0.01
43	12.2 ± 0.5	56 ± 2	0.22 ± 0.01
47	24 ± 1	82 ± 2	0.29 ± 0.02
48	57 ± 2	158 ± 4	0.36 ± 0.02
50	8.0 ± 0.4	21 ± 1	0.39 ± 0.03
51	11.2 ± 0.7	46 ± 3	0.24 ± 0.02
52	10.8 ± 0.8	46 ± 2	0.24 ± 0.02

Note: B—bronchus.
L—bronchopulmonary lymph node.
P—pleura of lung.
R—rib.
S—sternum.
V—vertebrae.
* Tumor present in sample analyzed.

first be discussed with respect to the concentrations of ^{210}Pb and ^{210}Po and their relationship to each other within specific body tissues.

Lung

Four different tissues from the pulmonary region were analyzed. Included are sections of the parenchyma, visceral pleura, bronchopulmonary lymph nodes and bronchus. Parenchymal samples were taken from the lung periphery and contained no bronchi larger than 1 mm in diameter. The visceral pleura was cut from the parenchymal tissue and included a small amount of the latter with associated lymphatic tissue. The two bronchi samples were from the region of the lower-lobe bronchus. In Table 2, B refers to bronchi, L to bronchopulmonary lymph node, P to visceral pleura, and no designation indicates parenchymal tissue.

The ^{210}Po and ^{210}Pb concentrations in the parenchymal tissues of the non-miners, 01–11, are, when compared to values in Table 3, very similar to concentrations which have been observed in "normal" lung tissue of smokers. Considering only tumor-free tissues, the concentrations of ^{210}Po and ^{210}Pb in all three pulmonary sample types were much greater in the miners than in the non-miners; as much as 300 times in the parenchymal tissue and 70 times in the lymph nodes. In nearly every case, ^{210}Po and ^{210}Pb were concentrated in the pleura relative to the parenchyma. The average activity in the pleura to that in the parenchyma was 1.6 for both ^{210}Po and ^{210}Pb. The same concentration effect is observed to occur in the lung of non-miners. This concentration of ^{210}Po and ^{210}Pb in the pleura is probably due to associated lymphatic tissue which tends to accumulate these nuclides and retain them for a longer period of time relative to the parenchymal tissue.

The lymph nodes contained the highest concentrations of ^{210}Po and ^{210}Pb of the pulmonary tissues. On the average, the ^{210}Pb concentration in the lymph nodes exceeded that in the parenchyma by nearly 4 times, with a maximum of 16 times. The concentrations of ^{210}Po and ^{210}Pb were the lowest in the bronchi specimens. Since it had been a number of years since these subjects had mined, nuclei deposited in the bronchus had undoubtedly long ago been cleared. The levels observed in these two bronchi samples are, however, significantly higher than an average value of 7.7 pCi ^{210}Po/kg. reported for 12 bronchi samples of non-exposed smokers.[14]

In all cases the ^{210}Po is supported by its ^{210}Pb parent. In the parenchyma the ^{210}Po/^{210}Pb activity ratio varied from 0.47 to 1.0 with an average of 0.72. In the pleura this ratio was only slightly higher, ranging from 0.61 to 0.95 with an average of 0.77.

Parenchymal tissue with associated tumor contained considerably less ^{210}Po and ^{210}Pb than did healthy adjacent tissue. Five samples of parenchymal tissue containing varying amounts of tumor were analyzed and the results compared with those of adjacent tissue having a normal appearance. The ratio of activities in tumor tissue/healthy tissue ranged from 0.10 to 0.42 for ^{210}Po and 0.16 to 0.44 for ^{210}Pb. No significant difference was noted in the affinity of the tumor for either ^{210}Po or ^{210}Pb, and the difference of concentration between the two samples appeared to be dependent solely on the amount of tumor present. This effect is also demonstrated by the tissues of miners 30, 38 and 41 in which the lymph nodes consisting of nearly all tumor contained smaller concentrations than did the parenchymal tissue. Hence, the concentrations measured in the lymph nodes of miners 37 and 50 which contain some tumor are suspect, even though they did contain higher levels than the parenchyma. These results emphasize the extreme care which must be exercised in selecting appropriate sample specimens for meaningful study.

Liver

The ^{210}Po and ^{210}Pb levels in the liver of miners exceeds by many times the liver concentrations which have previously been reported for unexposed individuals and listed in Table 3, while liver concentrations of the latter are similar to those observed in the non-miners, 02 and 11. The average ^{210}Po/^{210}Pb activity ratio in the miners' liver is 1.3 ± 0.5, which is

171

Table 3. Concentrations of ^{210}Pb–^{210}Po in tissues of unexposed adult populations as given in other reports

Tissue†	^{210}Po (pCi/kg)	^{210}Pb (pCi/kg)	Reference
Liver	14.5 (5–27)	9.2 (3–18)	7
	18.5		6
		8.8	17
Kidney	11.3 (3–25)	4.3 (2–12)	7
	18.5		6
		5	17
Lung	3.2, 10* (1–5)	5.6, 8.4* (0.6–10)	7
	1.5, 7.4* (2–23)*		11
	3.8, 10*		6
		(4.3–10)* 1.5, 6.1*	12
Spleen	3.5 (1.4–6.8)	3.7 (1–11)	7
		3.0	17
	6.6	7.5 (4–10)	7
Testes	3.9 (3.6–6.6)		6
Muscle		2.7	17
Heart	0.5 (0.4–0.6) (2–9)	0.4 (0.2–0.6)	7
Peribronchial lymph nodes	6.0, 11.6* (3–34)*		11
Thyroid	5.4 (2–13)	7.7 (2.4–15)	7
		161	18
Bone	(21–180) 90, 250* (67–600)*	(67–453) 135, 285* (178–502)*	12
		118	17
		1.4	17
Blood	(0.25–2.8) 0.76, 1.72* (0.6–4.8)*		13

* Indicates cigarette smokers.
† Soft tissue results refer to fresh wt. and bone results refer to ash wt.

smaller but not significantly different from the average ratio of 1.9 ± 0.3 reported for unexposed individuals.[7]

Nine samples of liver tissue containing varying amounts of tumor were also analyzed and compared to adjacent tissue having a normal appearance. The ratio of activities in tumor tissue to healthy tissue ranged from 0.17 to 0.89 for ^{210}Po and 0.09–0.87 for ^{210}Pb. Tissue containing the larger percentages of tumor had the lower ratios. For example, the minimum ratios of 0.17 and 0.09 refer to pure liver tumor, while the 0.89 and 0.87 ratios refer to tissue containing about 10% tumor. As in lung tissue, the ^{210}Po/^{210}Pb ratios did not show any affinity of the tumor for one nuclide relative to the other.

Kidney

The cortex and medulla of the kidney were analyzed separately, and the concentrations listed in Table 2 are those found in the cortex, by far the larger of the two sections. The levels observed in the kidneys of the non-miners, 02 and 11, fall within the range of values which have been reported for unexposed individuals as listed in Table 3, whereas, the levels found in the kidney of the miners, particularly ^{210}Po, are much greater. In all cases, the ^{210}Po activity was greater in the cortex than its ^{210}Pb parent, and the ^{210}Po/^{210}Pb activity ratio varied from 1.9 to 25, with an average of 8.6. The higher ratios generally occurred with the higher ^{210}Po concentrations and radon daughter exposures. The average ratio observed in the kidney cortex of miners is significantly greater than the 2.9 ^{210}Po/^{210}Pb ratio reported for the kidney of an unexposed population.[7] This shows a strong preference by the cortex of the kidney for the absorption of ^{210}Po.

In all cases, the medulla of the kidney contained less ^{210}Po than did the cortex, reflecting a nonuniform distribution within the kidney. The ^{210}Po(cortex)/^{210}Po(medulla) ratio ranged from 1.4 to 10 with an average of 4.2 ± 2.2. Also, the average ^{210}Po/^{210}Pb activity ratio in the medulla was 2.5 ± 0.9 and significantly less than the average ratio found in the cortex. In the case of ^{210}Pb, the ratio, ^{210}Pb(cortex)/^{210}Pb(medulla), ranged from 0.80 to 3.2, with an average of 1.5 ± 0.6. Consequently, ^{210}Po is concentrated to a much greater extent in the cortex than in the medulla, whereas, there does not appear to be any preferential absorption of ^{210}Pb. As one might expect, the ^{210}Po concentration and the ^{210}Po/^{210}Pb ratio observed in the cortical-medullary junction fell between the values found in the cortex and medulla portions of the kidney.

Spleen

The spleen was selected for study because phagocytosis, a function of the spleen, may tend to concentrate certain trace elements from the blood supply. The results show a higher concentration of both ^{210}Po and ^{210}Pb than the values which have been reported for unexposed individuals shown in Table 3. The spleen ranks third, behind lung and liver, in ^{210}Pb concentration of the analyzed soft tissues. The ratio of the concentration of ^{210}Po and ^{210}Pb in the spleen of miners to that observed in normal tissue range from about 2–50 times and 3–60 times, respectively. In all cases, the ^{210}Po is supported by its ^{210}Pb parent, and normally the ^{210}Pb is present in considerable excess, as reflected by an average ^{210}Po/^{210}Pb activity ratio of 0.49, the smallest observed in all tissues studied. This small ratio is probably in part a consequence of the even smaller ratio observed in blood (see below).

Only one tumor was observed in the spleen samples, and that in miner No. 48. The tumor contained only 47 % of the radionuclide concentration observed in the healthy portion of the sample.

Testis

The testis is a tissue which has been observed to concentrate ^{210}Po.[19] In all cases, the ^{210}Po/^{210}Pb activity ratio of the testes exceeds one, and the mean ratio for the miners is 4.8 ± 2.1. The ^{210}Po concentration exceeded that normally observed in testes of unexposed individuals by as much as 30 times.

The two testes were analyzed separately and found not to contain significantly different concentrations. The average of the two analyses are the concentrations given in Table 2.

Four samples of epididymis and tunica albuginea were also analyzed and the results compared to those for the testis. The epididymis and tunica albuginea contained much less ^{210}Po than the testis, 46% and 25% respectively. The opposite was true for ^{210}Pb, however, as the epididymis and tunica albuginea contained on the average 3.2 and 4.0 times respectively, that which was measured in the testis.

Muscle and heart

The concentrations of ^{210}Po and ^{210}Pb are similar in muscle and in the heart, and in both, the ^{210}Po is generally supported by ^{210}Pb. Although the ^{210}Po/^{210}Pb activity ratios are variable, the average does not significantly differ from one. The concentrations in the heart and muscle are low relative to the other soft tissues of the miners, although, they were generally higher than concentrations which have been observed in similar tissues of unexposed individuals. No difference in concentrations were observed in the heart between the right ventricular wall, the interventricular septum or the left ventricular wall.

Other soft tissues

Lymph node samples 11, 20, 26, 28, 44 and 47 were taken from the upper abdomen and all were anthracotic. Samples 13, 18, 24, 30, 33, 48 and 50 were parapancreatic lymph nodes while sample 54 was a paraortic lymph node. Typically, lymph nodes containing tumors, 13, 44 and 50, have smaller concentrations of ^{210}Po and ^{210}Pb. The lymph nodes are seen to concentrate both ^{210}Po and ^{210}Pb, however, the levels in these particular lymph nodes are considerably smaller than those observed above in the bronchopulmonary lymph nodes, a result of the avenue of exposure.

All small intestine samples were of the

175

duodenum, except sample No. 18 which was a segment of the illeum. The striking characteristic of these samples are the large $^{210}Po/^{210}Pb$ activity ratios. The activity ratios range from 1.6 to 2.7, with an average of 2.2. The concentrations in the stomach tissues are similar to those of the small intestine and also contain unsupported ^{210}Po.

The spinal cord contains relatively small concentrations of ^{210}Po and ^{210}Pb, with the ^{210}Po supported by the ^{210}Pb in each case. Brain was available from only one individual, and contained a higher activity of ^{210}Po than ^{210}Pb. The two brain samples, (a) the middle brain and (b) the medulla cortex, reflect no differences in concentration.

The samples of aorta contain surprisingly high concentrations. Sample No. 22 consisted of non-sclerotic tissue, while calcification was evident in sample No. 38. Atherosclerotic plaques, removed from the intima of samples No. 28 and No. 54, were analyzed separately and the results are designated as 28a and 54a. It is observed that ^{210}Po and ^{210}Pb concentrate in the atherosclerotic plaques, and that the concentrations in the aorta increase with calcification. Similar observations have been reported relative to high alpha activities and concentrations of ^{226}Ra and ^{210}Pb in calcified human aorta.[20,21]

Increased concentration with tissue calcification is evidenced in tissue other than the aorta. For example, the bronchopulmonary lymph node of miner No. 40 and the upper abdomenal lymph node of miner No. 47 were calcified and contain higher levels than might be expected from the concentrations in the other tissues of the same miners. Also, a calculis taken from miner No. 51 with 1.22% calcium contained 3.03 pCi $^{210}Po/g$ and 3.85 pCi $^{210}Pb/g$, which approaches the bone concentration. Hence, skeleton-seeking trace ions may be expected to concentrate when tissue calcification occurs.

Bone

The concentrations of ^{210}Po and ^{210}Pb in the bones of the non-miners, 02 and 11, are within

176

the range that has been reported for unexposed individuals as shown in Table 3. For the miners, concentrations are much greater. Using the average concentration of 161 pCi ^{210}Pb/kg ash reported by Holtzman for 83 individuals residing in the Chicago area,[18] and assuming the bone ash weight is 40% of fresh weight while defatted weight is 46% of fresh weight (see above),[22] the ash weight reported by Holtzman will be equivalent to about 140 pCi ^{210}Pb/kg of defatted bone. The ^{210}Pb concentrations in the rib samples of the uranium miners range from 2 to more than 40 times this average value.

The mean ^{210}Po/^{210}Pb activity ratio for the rib and vertebra are 0.77 ± 0.18 (S.D.) and 0.75 ± 0.11 (S.D.), respectively. Similar activity ratios were obtained for the two sternum samples. Except for samples 13 and 20, the concentrations observed in the rib to those in the vertebra are similar. The average ratios for ^{210}Po and ^{210}Pb in rib to that in the vertebra are 0.98 ± 0.25 and 1.04 ± 0.30 (S.D.), respectively. These results indicate that the concentrations of ^{210}Po and ^{210}Pb in various bones of the skeleton may not differ greatly, and that a reasonable estimate of skeletal burden can probably be achieved with the analysis of one bone type.

As in soft tissues, tumorous bone tissue contained less ^{210}Po and ^{210}Pb than was present in adjacent healthy tissue. Comparisons were made between three samples of bone tumor and healthy tissue. The average ^{210}Po and ^{210}Pb fractions remaining in the tumor tissue were about the same in each bone type; 34% in the rib and 22% in the vertebra.

Blood

The only blood sample available from a non-miner, 11, contained levels similar to those given in Table 3 for unexposed individuals. Concentrations in the blood of the miners were elevated and show a significantly greater ^{210}Pb activity relative to ^{210}Po. The mean ^{210}Po/^{210}Pb activity ratio of the 16 blood samples was calculated to be 0.35 ± 0.13 (S.D.), with a range of 0.22–0.73.

DISCUSSION

The concentration of ^{210}Pb in bone has been shown to increase with increased radon daughter exposures.[1,2] A correlation coefficient of 0.89 was reported for exposure vs. ^{210}Pb bone concentration when a correction was applied to account for ^{210}Pb excretion during the time interval of exposure to death.[2] Concentrations of ^{210}Pb in other body tissues do not appear to correlate well with exposure, although the concentrations of both ^{210}Pb and ^{210}Po in soft tissues do appear to be influenced to a large degree by the concentration in the skeleton. If the concentration in soft tissues is compared with the concentration in bone, a linear correlation is observed to exist in a number of cases. Excluding miners who have been exposed within a year of their death, linear correlation coefficients were calculated and are tabulated below. For ^{210}Pb:

	R	P
bone vs. liver	0.65	0.01
bone vs. lung	0.60	0.01
bone vs. spleen	0.82	<0.005

For ^{210}Po:

bone vs. liver	0.64	<0.025
bone vs. kidney	0.75	0.005
bone vs. testes	0.75	<0.005

For individuals who have not been exposed for a few months, the skeletal reservoir appears to become the most significant source of ^{210}Po and ^{210}Pb for other body compartments. Soft tissues will be continually resupplied with these nuclides and their burdens will not decrease with their assigned effective half-lives. For an active miner, the tissue concentrations will be influenced by both the skeletal burden and the atmospheric exposure.

Concentrations of ^{210}Pb and ^{210}Po in the various body tissues relative to that in liver are listed in Table 4 in the order of decreasing ^{210}Po levels. Tissues with associated tumors or lymph nodes which were calcified were

178

Table 4. *Mean concentrations relative to liver and percent body burden of* ^{210}Po *and* ^{210}Pb *in various tissues*

Tissue	^{210}Po Relative concentration*	^{210}Po %BB	^{210}Pb Relative concentration*	^{210}Pb %BB
Rib	11.8 ± 1.2‡	76.7	19.5 ± 3.4‡	78.7
Vertebra	12.7 ± 1.3‡		17.3 ± 1.6‡	
Lymph nodes, pulmonary	7.4 ± 3.7	1.4	11.8 ± 3.5	1.6
Lungs, parenchyma	2.8 ± 0.7	5.6	3.7 ± 0.9	4.9
Lymph nodes (other)	2.5 ± 0.7	2.9	3.6 ± 1.1	2.8
Kidney	2.2 ± 0.2	1.3	0.37 ± 0.06	0.2
Liver	1.00	3.3	1.00	2.2
Testes	0.37 ± 0.03	0.02	0.13 ± 0.02	0.01
Adrenal gland	0.34 ± 0.08	0.01	0.08 ± 0.01	<0.01
Spleen	0.27 ± 0.06	0.08	0.70 ± 0.16	0.2
Small intestine	0.24 ± 0.07	0.5	0.13 ± 0.03	0.2
Pancreas	0.19 ± 0.03	0.03	0.16 ± 0.06	0.01
Stomach	0.14 ± 0.02	0.07	0.11 ± 0.01	0.04
Brain	0.14	0.4	0.04	0.08
Thyroid	0.13	0.01	0.07	<0.01
Prostate	0.10 ± 0.02	<0.01	0.16 ± 0.05	<0.01
Spinal cord	0.09 ± 0.01	0.01	0.27 ± 0.10	0.01
Heart	0.08 ± 0.01	0.05	0.08 ± 0.01	0.03
Blood	0.08 ± 0.01	0.8	0.22 ± 0.02	1.6
Muscle	0.07 ± 0.01	4.1	0.11 ± 0.03	4.4
Other tissue†	—	2.3	—	3.0

* Concentrations in pCi relative to liver equated to 1.00.

† Concentrations assumed equal to that in muscle.

‡ Based on defat weight.

% BB = the per cent of the total body burden contained in organ of reference.

179

omitted, and the skeletal values refer to defatted bone. The uncertainties shown are the standard deviations of the mean. In all cases insufficient samples were available to show a definite normal distribution, and frequency plots of the relative concentrations indicate a possible positive skewness. Hence, the standard deviations may not include all information necessary to describe the population, and additional samples for this purpose would have been desirable.

The relative concentrations of ^{210}Po are normally less variable for a particular tissue than that of ^{210}Pb, however, the relative concentration of both nuclides do not vary greatly as shown by the standard deviations. This would indicate that generally the distribution in the body of ^{210}Po or ^{210}Pb is similar among individuals of a population group. In the case of some tissues, however, differences are noted between this population group and unexposed individuals.[7] Especially significant are the much higher relative concentrations of ^{210}Po and ^{210}Pb found in the lungs, and ^{210}Po found in the kidney of the miner population. Consequently, relative distribution within the body may change upon exposure, and differences may also occur with the avenue of exposure. For example, in the Alaskan caribou eating population that ingests larger than normal amounts of ^{210}Po, the concentration in the lung relative to the liver is much smaller than in the uranium miner.[23]

Also shown in Table 4 is the per cent of the total body burden for each tissue measured. These fractional body burdens were determined by multiplying the relative concentration of each organ by its mass, using the values listed by ICRP for the standard 70 kg man,[24] and determining the fraction of each to the sum in all tissues. Assuming a 70 kg man, the contents of ^{210}Pb and ^{210}Po in 71 % of the body mass can be directly estimated from the measurements. In the remaining 29%, the concentrations of ^{210}Po and ^{210}Pb were assumed equivalent to muscle. Although the concentration in some of the unanalyzed tissues may exceed that in muscle, about 50% of this tissue consists of fat which probably contains a somewhat smaller concentration than muscle, hence, using the concentration in muscle is probably a reasonable estimate. The skeletal mass was considered to be 3220 g defat weight (7000 g fresh weight × 0.46).

It is seen that by far the largest amount of ^{210}Po and ^{210}Pb in the body is contained in the skeleton (~78%). The value for ^{210}Pb is in good agreement with those reported by Osborne, 80%[25] and Stahlhofen, 70%,[26] and between the 63% reported by Holtzman[27] and the 90% reported by Black.[29] Fractional ^{210}Pb body burdens reported by Holtzman and Osborne for the liver, spleen, kidney and blood are in very close agreement with those shown in Table 4, however, they both report a per cent muscle burden of about 3 times that reported here.[25,27] The fractional body burden of ^{210}Po in the skeleton has been estimated as 80% by Osborne and 61% by Stahlhofen.[25,28] The lower value in the latter case is partially explained by a higher relative muscle concentration which he applied to 44% of the body mass that was not analyzed. Since the muscle concentration has been applied to a substantial portion of the body mass, some disagreement may be expected in addition to differences which might arise as a consequence of exposure. For both nuclides, then, the skeleton is the major reservoir in the body, while in the soft tissue category, the lymph nodes, lung, liver and muscle contain the largest quantities. The kidney should be considered an important reservoir for ^{210}Po, and possibly the blood for ^{210}Pb.

The body burdens of ^{210}Po and ^{210}Pb were calculated for those miners whose tissues that were analyzed represented more than 60% of the body mass and, as seen from Table 4, probably more than 90% of the body burden. The body burden for each miner was estimated by summing the concentrations observed in each tissue multiplied by the tissue mass.[24] As before, the concentration in tissue not determined was assumed to be the same as that found in the muscle and was based on the 70 kg "standard man". The estimated body burdens of ^{210}Po and ^{210}Pb for 19 uranium miners and 2 non-miners at the time of death are given in Table 5.

The body burden of ^{210}Po calculated for the two non-miners agrees with a value of 0.49 nCi estimated by STAHLHOFEN for an unexposed population.[28] JAWOROWSKI estimates that the ^{210}Pb body burden of residents in the Northern Temperate Zone is about 0.40 nCi.[17] This estimate may be a little low in view of ^{210}Pb skeletal and soft tissue results reported by HOLTZMAN and BLANCHARD which indicate a ^{210}Pb body burden in the order of 0.50–0.55 nCi, similar to that reported for non-miners in Table 5.[18,7] The estimated body burdens for the miners varied from 1.6 nCi to 22.8 nCi of ^{210}Po and from 2.3 nCi to 33.3 nCi of ^{210}Pb. These burdens range from about 4 to 50 times the burdens observed for the non-miners. It is also seen that the body burden of ^{210}Pb exceeds that for ^{210}Po in every case, and the average value of the ratio ^{210}Po body burden/^{210}Pb body burden is 0.74 $\pm$ 0.09 (S.D.), very similar to the ratio for the non-miners.

The fraction of ^{210}Po in the organ of reference to that in the total body (f_2) and the maximum permissible body burden (MPBB) as given by ICRP are compared in Table 6 to values calculated from data obtained in this study.[30] With respect to bone, the MPBB is based on a comparison with 0.1 μCi ^{226}Ra, and calculated as shown by ICRP using a relative damage factor for ^{210}Po of 5.[31] It is seen from this table that considerable differences exist between values reported by ICRP and those calculated here. For the uranium miner population, the skeleton appears to be the critical organ for ^{210}Po and the MPBB in this case is 0.05 μCi. The same is probably true of other population groups whose body burden of ^{210}Po is mainly a result of ingrowth from internally deposited ^{210}Pb. Using a similar treatment for ^{210}Pb results in a MPBB of 0.5 μCi with the skeleton as the critical organ. This is due to an f_2 value of 0.79 instead of 0.56 as given by the ICRP.[30]

As seen from Table 5, the estimated ^{210}Pb body burdens are much less than the MPBB given above, the largest observed ^{210}Pb body

Table 5. *Uranium miner body burdens of* ^{210}Po *and* ^{210}Pb

Miner No.	At death			Estimated at end of mining	
	^{210}Po (nCi)	^{210}Pb (nCi)	^{210}Po/^{210}Pb	^{210}Po (nCi)	^{210}Pb (nCi)
13	1.6	2.4	0.67	3.6	4.7
18	2.5	3.4	0.74	13.8	18.7
20	5.5	8.0	0.69	8.1	11.7
22	3.4	6.0	0.57	5.1	9.1
24	1.9	2.3	0.82	5.0	6.0
26	6.3	7.5	0.84	18.1	21.5
28	5.4	6.6	0.82	7.9	9.7
29	—	13.7	—		26.7
33	11.5	17.8	0.65	18.2	28.1
36	12.7	16.0	0.79	18.7	23.5
38	16.3	27.1	0.60	16.3	27.1
40	6.5	7.7	0.84	30.1	35.7
44	7.3	11.7	0.62	33.2	59.1
45	4.7	5.2	0.90	8.0	56.8
47	19.7	24.9	0.79	51.4	74.8
48	22.8	33.3	0.69	36.0	52.5
51	15.5	18.6	0.83	27.4	32.8
52	10.1	13.0	0.78	23.9	30.8
53	14.5	19.5	0.74	16.4	26.4
Non-miners					
02	0.51	0.69	0.74		
11	0.41	0.57	0.72		

burden being only about 7% of the MPBB. For ^{210}Po, however, the body burden of some miners does not fall far below the above calculated MPBB of 0.05 μCi. The ^{210}Po body burdens observed range from 3 to 46% of this MPBB.

Table 6. *A comparison of ICRP values and calculated values of f_2 factors and maximum permissible body burdens,* ^{210}Po

Critical organ	ICRP*		Uranium miner results	
		MPBB		MPBB
	f_2	(μCi)	f_2	(μCi)
Bone†	0.08	0.5	0.77	0.05
Kidney	0.13	0.04	0.013	0.4
Liver	0.22	0.1	0.033	0.8
Spleen	0.07	0.03	0.0008	3.0
Lung	—	—	0.056	0.3

*Report of Committee II on permissible dose for internal radiation (1959), *Health Phys.* **3**, 12–15 (1960).
†Based on comparison with 0.1 μCi ^{226}Ra.

In addition, the body burdens observed at time of death are undoubtedly lower than when the miners were actively mining. Assuming the skeletal ^{210}Pb and ^{210}Po burden to be 75% of the body burden, and that the apparent effective half-life of ^{210}Po in the skeleton is the same as that for ^{210}Pb, the body burdens at the time the miners stopped mining may be estimated from the observed burdens by applying the following ^{210}Pb excretion equation derived by BLACK *et al.*[1]

$$R = R_0(0.25e^{-\lambda_1 T} + 0.75e^{-\lambda_2 T}) \qquad (1)$$

where: R = pCi ^{210}Pb/g at time of death
R_0 = pCi ^{210}Pb/g at time of last mining experience
λ_1 = 2.875 yr^{-1} (T_E = 88 days)
λ_2 = 0.1916 yr^{-1} (T_E = 1320 days)
T = time between last mining experience and death.

The body burdens at the time the miners stopped mining were estimated using equation

(1), and the results are given in Table 5. The estimated ^{210}Pb burdens are still far below the above calculated MPBB, however, the estimated ^{210}Po burdens now range from 7% to 103% of the calculated MPBB when the skeleton is taken as the critical organ. The average estimated body burden of ^{210}Po at the time the miners last left the mine is 21 nCi with one miner exceeding the calculated MPBB at that time.

The principal internal radiation dose to a uranium miner while actively mining is delivered to the lung by the short-lived radon-222 daughter products that are present in the mine atmosphere.[16,32] It has been estimated that a radon-222 daughter exposure of 1 WLM will deliver to bronchial tissue a dose of 7 ± 5 rads.[33] The radiation dose to other body tissues while actively mining, and to all body tissues during post mining periods, is due principally to the 5.3 MeV alpha emitter, ^{210}Po.

The dose contributed by a nuclide uniformly deposited in the mineral portion of the bone to the soft tissue within the cavities of the bone can be estimated according to SPEARS[34] and STAHLHOFEN[28] by the following equation,

$$D = 69.6c\Sigma n_{\gamma}\bar{E}_{\gamma}\bar{F}\ \text{rad/day} \qquad (2)$$

Table 7. *Radiation dose-rate from* ^{210}Po *to uranium miner tissues*

Tissue	Dose to miner Range	(mrad/ yr) Mean	Mean dose to non-miner (mrad/yr)
Bone	13–305	125	5.5
Liver	2–69	19	1.1
Kidney	3–150	34	1.7
Lung	1.2–138	47	0.5
Bronchopulmonary lymph node	16–171	70	2.4
Spleen	0.3–17	4	0.13
Testes	0.7–15	6	0.4
Lymph nodes	5.6–130	31	2

where $\Sigma n_\gamma \bar{E}_\gamma$ is the mean particle energy, 5.3 for ^{210}Po, F is the mean factor of geometry which converges to unity for very small dia. of the cavity, and c is the concentration in μCi/g. For the Haversian systems, the factor F for ^{210}Po has been calculated by STAHLHOFEN to be 1.0 for canaliculi of very small dia., 0.95 for osteocytes of 5μ dia. and 0.48 for Haversian canals of 50 μ dia.[28] Only the dose associated with canaliculi having an F value of 1.0 will be considered in this discussion.

The skeletal dose rates were calculated by equation (2) for each miner using the bone concentrations given in Table 2 multiplied by 0.46 (defat wt./fresh wt. ratio). The range and the average dose rate observed at death for the miners and the two non-miners are listed in Table 7. The skeletal dose from ^{210}Po to the miners ranged from about twice to more than 50 times that of the non-miners. Also the rad doses listed in Table 7 are an underestimate of the effective dose, since the RBE for the ^{210}Po alpha may be as high as 10, and has a relative damage factor of 5.[35] Hence, the skeletal dose rates at the time of death may have exceeded 15 rem/yr in some cases.

Considering the skeletal excretion of ^{210}Pb and ^{210}Po during the period between the last mining exposure and death, the dose rates listed in Table 7 are, in most cases, less than the dose rates during mining or shortly after the last mining exposure. Using equation (1) and assuming that the apparent effective half-lives of ^{210}Pb and ^{210}Po are similar in the skeleton, the average dose rate for these miners at the time of their last exposure is estimated to be 320 mrad/yr, with a maximum of 700 mrad/yr for miner No. 47. Assuming an RBE equal to 10 and a relative damage factor of 5, this is equivalent to about 35 rem/yr, exceeding that recommended by ICRP for an occupationally exposed population.[31] The infinite dose, (D_∞), is shown by Spears to be equal to 1.44 $D_0 T$; where D_0 is the dose rate at exposure and T is the effective half-life of the nuclide.[34] Assuming the effective half-life of ^{210}Po in the skeleton to be 1320 days (3.62 yr),[1] and taking D_0 as the dose rate at the time the miner stopped mining, the infinite dose which would be received by miner No. 47 is about 4 rads. This does not account for the dose which was delivered during the period of actual mining, and also, the infinite dose calculated may be conservative, as an effective half-life for ^{210}Pb on the order of 9 yr has been suggested.[27]

The skeletal dose delivered by ^{226}Ra appears to be small compared to the ^{210}Po dose. The concentrations of ^{226}Ra in rib samples of miners No. 48 and No. 34, determined by the emanation method described by LUCAS,[36] were 158 ± 17 pCi/kg and 51 ± 7 pCi/kg, respectively. Using equation (2) by setting F equal to 1.00 and $\Sigma n_y \bar{E}_y$ equal to 10.56 for ^{226}Ra and 30% of its short-lived decay products,[28] the dose absorbed is calculated to be 20 mrad/yr for sample No. 48 and 7 mrad/yr for sample No. 34. Hence, the dose rates associated with ^{226}Ra and its short-lived decay products are only about 7% of the ^{210}Po dose rates; 315 mrad/yr and 90 mrad/yr for the rib samples No. 48 and No. 34, respectively.

Assuming ^{210}Po to be evenly distributed in the soft tissues,[6] it can be shown that 1 pCi ^{210}Po/kg will deliver to the soft tissue 0.1 mrad/ yr. On this basis, the ^{210}Po dose delivered to the more important soft tissues were calculated and are listed in Table 7. Again taking the RBE to be equal to 10, all dose rates to individual soft tissues, although many times larger than the dose rates to tissues of unexposed individuals, are considerably less than the maximum permissible dose rate to individual organs set by ICRP for an occupationally exposed population.[37] One may only guess at what these soft-tissue dose rates were during the time of high exposure in a uranium mine, undoubtedly much higher; however, these values calculated at death would indicate that except for bone, the internal dose from ^{210}Po is below the maximum permissible exposure recommended by ICRP, and in all cases, is small compared to the estimated 7 ± 5 rad/ WLM delivered to the lung during mining by the short-lived radon daughter products.[33]

A previous report has suggested the possible existence of a correlation between the concentration of ^{210}Pb and ^{210}Po in bone and blood.[2] If a correlation does exist, it would be valuable as a means of estimating the body burden in living miners, and possibly in persons of other exposure groups as well. The ^{210}Pb blood concentrations are plotted with the rib concentrations in Fig. 1. The high blood concentration observed for sample 48, the circled point in Fig. 1, may be abnormal, as considerable tumor was found in both the rib and the vertebra. The rapid tumor may have released abnormally large amounts of ^{210}Pb and ^{210}Po from the skeleton. Tumorous tissue found in bone, as mentioned above, had less ^{210}Pb and ^{210}Po than was present in adjacent healthy bone tissue. The fraction remaining in the tumor tissue of this individual was 33% for the rib and 20% for the vertebra. Consequently, it is reasonable to assume that active bone tumors could cause an elevation in the blood concentration of ^{210}Pb and ^{210}Po. Disregarding, therefore, the sample of No. 48, the concentration of ^{210}Pb in blood increases linearly with the concentration of ^{210}Pb in the bone, and linear correlation coefficients calculated were 0.84 ($P < 0.001$) for the rib and 0.87 ($P < 0.001$) for the vertebra. The correlation with respect to ^{210}Po was not as high; $R = 0.73$ ($P = 0.001$) for the rib and $R = 0.79$ ($P = 0.001$) for the vertebra.

By the method of least squares analysis, the following equation was derived to describe the relationship between the concentration of ^{210}Pb in blood to that in the skeleton.

$$^{210}\text{Pb(pCi/g)bone}$$
$$= 0.58 + 0.0614(\text{pCi/kg})\text{blood} \quad (3)$$

The line of best-fit which is drawn through the points of Fig. 1, however, has been shifted slightly to pass through the origin, as the intercept was shown by the F Test to be statistically indistinguishable from zero. The equation of this linear regression line is:

$$^{210}\text{Pb(pCi/g)bone}$$
$$= 0.070(\text{pCi } ^{210}\text{Pb/kg})\text{blood} \quad (4)$$

Also shown in Fig. 1 are the 67% confidence limits on the individual observation. The per cent of deviation at the mean bone concentration is $\pm 40\%$. The arithmetic mean ratio, pCi/kg(blood)/pCi/g(bone), of ^{210}Pb is 16 ± 7 for the rib and 14 ± 4 for the vertebra. The uncertainties are the standard deviation of the ratios, which appear smaller in the case of the vertebra, and indicate that there is no difference between rib and vertebra. It should be mentioned that the ^{210}Pb data for bone and blood do not rule out the possibility of a log-normal distribution of the ratios. If this be the case, the geometric mean ratio for rib is $14 \overset{\times}{\div} 1.5$, and not a great deal different from the arithmetic mean ratio.

The ability to predict the skeletal burden of ^{210}Po from the blood concentration is more uncertain than in the case of ^{210}Pb. The mean blood/bone concentration ratios for ^{210}Po are 7 ± 4 for the rib and 7 ± 3 for the vertebra.

In addition to the correlations observed between the concentrations of ^{210}Pb and ^{210}Po in blood and bone, some soft tissue concentrations were observed to be correlated with the blood concentrations. The relationships that exhibited the higher linear correlations are tabulated below for ^{210}Po and ^{210}Pb along with the mean concentration ratios (C); pCi/kg(blood) $\div$ pCi/kg(tissue). The uncertainties shown are the standard deviation of the ratios.

^{210}Pb		R	P	C
	blood vs. liver	0.90	<0.001	0.23 ± 0.07
^{210}Po				
	blood vs. liver	0.90	<0.001	$8.5 \pm 2.7 \times 10^{-2}$
	blood vs. kidney	0.88	<0.001	$4.3 \pm 2.1 \times 10^{-2}$
	blood vs. spleen	0.83	0.001	0.44 ± 0.17

These data indicate that blood levels of ^{210}Pb and ^{210}Po do reflect their concentration in several body compartments. This may, however, be a special case, in which the skeleton is the major source of these nuclides to the blood and to other body organs. The blood concentration, regulated by the slow and steady release of these nuclides from the skeleton, remains fairly constant as do the smaller soft tissue reservoirs once equilibrium is established, and the apparent effective half-lives of ^{210}Pb and ^{210}Po in all

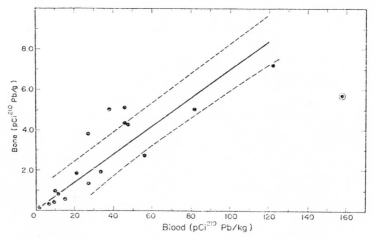

Fig. 1. The relationship of the ^{210}Pb concentration in blood to the concentration in bone with the 67% confidence limits on individual observations.

body compartments resembles that in the skeleton. From urine and bone data reported by BLACK *et al.*,[1] it appears that after a final exposure it will require from 3 to 6 months for this equilibrium within the body to be established. When exposure is resumed, the equilibrium between skeleton-blood-soft tissue will be disrupted due to increased blood and soft tissue levels, and the blood/tissue correlations observed here will no longer exist.

SUMMARY

(1) Concentrations of [210]Po and ^{210}Pb are higher in tissues of uranium miners and in some cases much higher, approaching 300 times in lung parenchyma, than in tissues of an unexposed population.

(2) For the principal body compartments containing [210]Po, the fractions of the total body burden were observed to be: skeleton, 77%; lung, 5.6%; lymph nodes, 4.3%; muscle, 4%; and kidney, 1.3%. For ^{210}Pb, the major fractional body burdens were found to be the skeleton, 79%; lungs, 4.9%; muscle, 4.4%;

lymph nodes, 4.4%; liver, 2.2%; and blood, 1.6%. The results also indicate that generally the relative distribution in the body of ^{210}Pb and ^{210}Po is similar among individuals in a population group, however, differences in the relative body distribution were noted between the miner population and the unexposed population. In the case of some tissues, the relative body distribution may also change with the avenue of exposure.

(3) Estimated body burdens of the miners at death varied from 1.6 nCi to 22.8 nCi for ^{210}Po and from 2.3 nCi to 33.3 nCi for ^{210}Pb, with a mean $^{210}Po/^{210}Pb$ body ratio of 0.74 ± 0.09 (S.D.). This ratio is very similar to that observed in non-miners.

(4) The dose rates delivered by ^{210}Po to the soft tissues fell well below the maximum permissible limit recommended by the ICRP, however, the maximum permissible limit of 30 rem/yr for bone may have been exceeded in some cases. The ^{210}Po dose in all cases, however, is probably small compared to the estimated 7 ± 5 rad/WLM delivered during mining to the bronchial tissue of the lung by the short-lived radon daughter products.

(5) Tissues with tumor contained less ^{210}Po and ^{210}Pb than adjacent healthy tissue, emphasizing the care with which tissues must be selected for study.

(6) Increased ^{210}Po and ^{210}Pb concentrations are observed to occur upon soft tissue calcification; for example, aorta, lymph nodes, etc.

(7) Good correlations were observed between the ^{210}Pb concentration in blood to that in bone and liver, while for ^{210}Po, good correlations were observed between the concentration in blood to that in bone, liver, kidney, and spleen. The results suggest the possibility of utilizing blood concentrations as an index to the body burden of these nuclides, especially of ^{210}Pb.

(8) The uranium miner population may be unique, as after a miner has had no exposure for a number of months, the skeletal reservoir becomes the most important source of ^{210}Pb and ^{210}Po for the other body compartments. An equilibrium is established between skeleton-

blood-soft tissue, with the consequence that the effective half-lives of both ^{210}Pb and ^{210}Po in blood and the soft-tissue compartments are similar to that for ^{210}Pb in the skeleton.

Acknowledgements—The authors thank Dr. G. SACCO-MANNO, St. Mary's Hospital, Grand Junction, and Dr. OSCAR AUERBACH, Veterans Administration Hospital, East Orange, for the tissue specimens, Dr. RICHARD SWARM, Cincinnati University School of Medicine, who sectioned and examined the tissue specimens, Dr. V. E. ARCHER and C. M. PHELAN, Occupational Health Field Station, Salt Lake City, who furnished the exposure data and mining histories, and of this laboratory, Dr. BERND KAHN whose suggestions were very helpful throughout the study.

REFERENCES

1. S. C. BLACK, V. E. ARCHER, W. C. DIXON and G. SACCOMANNO, *Health Phys.* **14,** 81 (1968).
2. R. L. BLANCHARD, V. E. ARCHER and G. SAC-COMANNO, *Health Phys.* **16,** 585 (1969).
3. Z. S. JAWOROWSKI, *Atompraxis* **11,** 271 (1965).
4. R. L. BLANCHARD, *Nature, Lond.* **223,** 287 (1969).
5. E. POHL, Dose distribution received on inhalation of ^{222}Rn and its Decay products. *Radiological Health and Safety in Mining and Milling of Nuclear Materials,* Vol. I. IAEA, Vienna, 221 (1964).
6. C. R. HILL, *Nature, Lond.* **208,** 423 (1965).
7. R. L. BLANCHARD, *Health Phys.* **13,** 625 (1967).
8. K. Z. MORGAN, W. S. SNYDER and M. R. FORD, *Health Phys.* **10,** 151 (1964).
9. A. MARTIN, *Health Phys.* **13,** 1348 (1967).
10. S. C. BLACK, *Health Phys.* **7,** 87 (1961).
11. J. B. LITTLE, E. P. RADFORD, H. L. McCOMBS and V. R. HUNT, *N. Engl. J. Med.* **273,** 1343 (1965).
12. R. B. HOLTZMAN and F. H. ILCEWICZ, *Science* **153,** 1259 (1966).
13. J. B. LITTLE and R. B. McGANDY, *Nature, Lond.* **211,** 842 (1966).
14. B. RAJEWSKY and W. STAHLHOFEN, *Nature, Lond.* **209,** 1312 (1966).
15. V. E. ARCHER and C. M. PHELAN, personal communication (1969).
16. Public Health Service Publication No. 494: *Control of Radon and Radon Daughters in Uranium Mines and Calculation of Biological Effects,* U.S. Department of Health, Education and Welfare (1956).
17. Z. S. JAWOROWSKI, *Stable and Radioactive Lead*

in Environment and Human Body, Inst. of Nucl. Res., Nucl. Energy Inf. Center, Warsaw (1967).

18. R. B. HOLTZMAN, *Health Phys.* **9**, 385 (1963).
19. L. D. SAMUELS, *Nature, Lond.* **210**, 434 (1966).
20. A. ELKELES, *Br. J. Radiol.* **34**, 602 (1961).
21. N. COHEN, personal communication (1967).
22. R. B. HOLTZMAN, *Health Phys.* **8**, 315 (1962).
23. R. L. BLANCHARD and J. B. MOORE, *Health Phys.* **18**, 127 (1970).
24. Report of Committee II on permissible dose for internal radiation, *Health Phys.* **3**, 151 (1960).
25. R. V. OSBORNE, *Nature, Lond.* **199**, 295 (1963).
26. W. STAHLHOFEN, personal communication (1964).
27. R. B. HOLTZMAN, ANL-6297 (1960).
28. W. STAHLHOFEN, *Assessment of Radioactivity in Man*, p. 505. IAEA, Vienna (1964).
29. S. C. BLACK, *AMA Archs envir. Hlth* **5**, 423 (1962).
30. Report of Committee II on permissible dose for internal radiation, *Health Phys.* **3**, 75 and 217 (1960).
31. Report of Committee II on permissible dose for internal radiation, *Health Phys.* **3**, 12 (1960).
32. Guidance for the Control of Radiation Hazards in Uranium Mining, FRC Rep. No. 8, 60 pp., September (1967).
33. Radiation exposure of uranium miners, Rep. Advis. Comm. Div. Med. Sci.: Nat. Acad. Sci.—Nat. Res. Coun.—Nati. Acad. Engng, Washington, D.C., 31 pp., August (1968).
34. F. W. SPEARS, Dosimetry of radioisotopes in soft tissues and in bone. *Proc. Enrico Fermi Int. School Phys.; Radiation Dosimetry* (Edited by G. W. REED), p. 269. Academic Press, New York (1964).
35. Report of Committee II on permissible dose for internal radiation, *Health Phys.* **3**, 29 (1960).
36. H. F. LUCAS, ANL-6297, 55 (1961).
37. Report of Committee II on permissible dose for internal radiation, *Health Phys.* **3**, 4 (1960).

Ulcer and Gastritis in the Professions Exposed to Lead

Brana Jovičić

THERE ARE still gaps in our knowledge of the genesis of lead poisoning. Factors of inheritance and physical and chemical toxic influences do not present adequate answers. Research is still needed, and efforts of research workers throughout the world should be pooled.

The impact of lead in the pathogenesis of ulcer has been the subject of extensive research which has involved different interpretations and conclusions. In 1921, Glaser[1] found 12 ulcers among 21 cases of lead poisoning. In 1919, Schiff[2] announced that ulcer is found more often among workers in contact with lead. Glaser[1] and Lewis[3] believed that ulcer and gastroenteritis are more frequent among employees handling lead. Kapp[4] reported increased frequency of ulcer in lead workers.

Gray[5] found that 10% of 150 workers exposed to lead had duodenal ulcers. All of these cases had existing ulcers which were aggravated as a result of lead intoxication. Gray also pointed out some cases of his own which were aggravated as a direct consequence of lead intoxication. He also described the case of a patient, a painter for many years, who had lead intoxications but who, at autopsy, had marked changes in cerebral blood vessels but no ulcer.

In a group of 268 patients with lead poisoning, Bellini and Finulli[6] reported 18 patients, or 3.9%, with ulcer compared to the control group in whom the percentage was 1.15.

Many other authors, both Eastern and Western, have denied the importance of lead in the pathogenesis of ulcer. The best-documented studies are certainly those of des Planches[7] and Csepai.[8] In des Planches' study, only 12, or 1.2%, of 1,000 workers who worked with lead had ulcer. Csepai had complete documentation from an insurance society at his disposal; he reported no correlation between ulcer and lead. Soviet authors Makaritschewa and Glagolewa[9] agree with Csepai, Vernetti[10] and Gutzert,[11] quoted by Cordet,[12] believe that the appearance of ulcer in cases of lead intoxication is an exceptional rarity.

Cordet,[12] who devoted his dissertation to this question, found only two lead workers in a group of 225 ulcer patients; neither of these showed signs of lead intoxication.

Mechanism of Action

Although the histological picture of tissues of persons chronically intoxicated by lead is not pathognomonic, in contrast to the situation in acute intoxication, there is a belief that lead, in those constantly exposed to it, causes spasm of the capillaries of the pylorus and duodenal bulb with ischemia and atrophy of the mucosa. Some authors do not exclude a direct toxic action of lead on the duodenal mucosa. Injuries to the walls of blood vessels as well as the more frequent toxic vagatomy caused by lead are mentioned as etiological factors in ulcer.[6,13]

The aim of our work is to try to define the relationship between exposure to lead and ulcer and gastritis, as well as to gastric acidity.

Procedure

For 2½ years we have singled out patients with confirmed diagnoses of peptic ulcer, gastritis, and saturnism and presaturnism. All patients suffering from ulcers had radiological confirmation of their diagnosis. Gastritis was accepted on the basis of symptomatology and radiological appearance. The diagnosis of lead intoxication was based on history of occupational exposure, subjective symptomatology, and laboratory analyses (basophilic stippling of erythrocytes, coproporphyrinuria). Diagnosis of saturnism was established according to information about length of exposure as well as the classic symptomatology, lead colic, anemia, and increased lead values in the blood (over $100\gamma/100$ cu cm) and coproporphyrin in urine over $150\gamma/liter$ (Baker's method; upper limit of normal 60 to $80\gamma/100\%$. Coproporphyrin in urine by the method of Askevold upper limit, $120\gamma/liter$ of urine in 24 hours).

The diagnosis of presaturnism was based on exposure data as well as on symptomatological characteristic of the early stage of plumbism without anemia or colic; lead values and cor-

proporphyrin were increased after provocation with calcium ethylenediaminetetracetic acid. In the control group of patients with gastritis, all patients with this diagnosis were accepted unless they had lead or another intoxication. Efforts were made to obtain comparable age and socioeconomic groups. Gastric acidity was studied by fractional analysis, using caffeine.

Findings

Group With Ulcer.—Of 112 patients with confirmed ulcer, presaturnism was confirmed in 14, or 12.5%. Ulcer was localized to the duodenum in ten cases, and four had gastric ulcer.

The group with saturnism numbered 35 patients and with presaturnism, 125. Of this number, gastric radiography had been done on only 103, 21 with saturnism and 82 with presaturnism. Of this group, 88, or 85.3%, had a diagnosis of gastritis. Of 21 patients with saturnism, 18, or 85.6%, had confirmed gastritis while in the group of 82 patients with presaturnism, 70, or 85.5%, were confirmed. No patient with saturnism had ulcer.

In the same group, gastric acidity was studied in 68 patients, of which 14 had saturnism and 54 presaturnism. Hypoacidic values were found in all patients with saturnism while hypoacidic values in the group of patients with presaturnism were no free acid in six patients, hypoacidity in 38, or 56%, hyperacidity in four, and normal acidity in six. Hypoacidity was found in 76.5% of all cases and in 70.6% of the 54 patients with presaturnism.

The control group of 94 patients had the following values: hypoacidity, 51, or 54.3%; normal acidity, 38; and no free acid, 5.

Age.—The age of patients with saturnism and presaturnism is shown in the following tabulation:

21 to 30	33
31 to 40	50
41 to 50	13
51 to 60	8
Total	103

The length of exposure to lead ranged from 12 months to 35 years.

Only two patients with ulcer and ten patients with gastric disease reported previous digestive disturbances.

195

Occupation.—The greatest number, 39, of those exposed to lead had worked with storage batteries (as lubricators, cutters, joining and forming storage battery blocks). Other workers were welders, foundry workers, potters, painters, and varnishers.

Comment

The frequency of ulcer in the general population of Yugoslavia varies from 3% to 15%, according to Han[14] and Jovičić.[15] The figure of 12.5% for those exposed to lead does not permit firm conclusions to be drawn that there is a relationship between lead exposure and ulcer.

Negligible differences in the prevalence of ulcer between control and exposed groups, 1.15% and 3.9%, as reported by Bellini and Finulli,[6] cannot serve as proof that lead is a factor in the appearance of peptic ulcer, especially since the prevalence of ulcer in various populations is not known. As a matter of fact, the prevalence of ulcer is known to vary in various parts of the same country.

Specific information about the high frequency of gastritis has greater importance, especially the important differences in gastric acidity. Hypoacidity was present in 76.5% of those exposed to lead. There was an important difference in hypoacidity of 22.2% between the exposed and the control group which suggests with greater certainty the impact of lead on gastric secretion.

References

1. Glaser A: Ulzerrationen im Magen-Darmkanal und chronische Bleivergiftung. *Berlin Klin Wschr* 4:111-152, 1921.

2. Schiff AM: Chronischer Saturnismus bei Ulcus ventriculi und vegetatives Nervensystem. *Wien Klin Wschr* 32:387-390, 1919.

3. Lewis DR: Lead poisoning as a cause of peptic ulcer. *Brit Med J* 1:185-188, 1932.

4. Kapp H: Ulcus duodeni als Unfallserkrankung. *Gastroenterologia* 64:290-298, 1939.

5. Gray IJ: Gastrointestinal disease in relation to occupational hazards. *Gastroenterology* 4:61-71, 1945.

6. Bellini F, Finulli M: Gastroduodenite et ulcera peptica nel saturnismo. *Med Lavoro* 51:369-372, 1960.

7. des Planches T: *Traité des Maladies du Plomb.* Paris, 1939, vol 1 and 2.

8. Csepai K: Bleivergiftung und Magengeschwür. *Mschr Unfallheilk* 45:425-428, 1938.

9. Makaritschewa A, Glagolewa T: Ulcus of the stomach in lead workers. *J Industr Hyg* 16:201-205, 1934.

10. Vernetti BL: Saturnismo cronico ed ulcera gastroduodenale. *Med Lavoro* 24:216-221, 1933.

11. Gutzert KL: Les lésions de la muqueuse gastrique chez les saturniens. *München Med Wschr* 21:9014, 1928.

12. Cordet ME: *Contribution à l'étude de l'étiologie professionnelle de l'ulcère gastro-duodénal chez i'homee,* thesis. Lyon, France, 1963.

13. Beeson BP, McDermott W: *Textbook of Medicine,* ed 11. Philadelphia and London, WB Saunders Co, 1963, pp 2115-2120.

14. Han A: Gastro-duodenalni ulcus. *Lijech Vjesn* 4:365-385, 1961.

15. Jovičić DB: *Gastro-duodenal Ulcer in Serbien,* thesis. Belgrade, Yugoslavia, 1968.

Methods For Analytical Detection Of Lead

TECHNICAL NOTE

MICRODETERMINATION OF LEAD ON TAPES OF AN A.I.S.I. AUTOMATIC AIR SAMPLER BY ATOMIC ABSORPTION SPECTROSCOPY

W. A. M. DEN TONKELAAR
MARTHA A. BIKKER

INTRODUCTION

To ESTABLISH hygienic and legal standards for the prevention and control of air pollution it is necessary to make prolonged, continuous investigations of the nature, quantity and fluctuations of the various contaminants.

The purpose of this study is to develop a simple, fast and very sensitive routine method for the determination of lead in airborne particulates.

To correlate the particulate lead concentration with time of day, traffic density and meteorological conditions, 2-h samples were collected on a continuous tape sampler. This method of collection was also used by CHOLAK *et al.* (1961) and DIGGS *et al.* (1963) to determine diurnal fluctuations in the concentration of lead compounds. Atomic absorption spectroscopy provides a simple technique for the analysis of metals and its feasibility for determining the lead content of particulate matter has already been demonstrated by BULLOCK and LEWIS (1968), BURNHAM *et al.* (1969) and CHOLAK *et al.* (1969).

In a comparison study of the dithizone and atomic absorption methods of determining lead in airborne particulates a correlation coefficient of 0·996 was found (HELLER, 1969).

The present technique has been performed on samples taken during 1968 and 1969 and will be continued to provide more definitive data on levels and trends of atmospheric lead.

EXPERIMENTAL

Apparatus

Analyses were carried out with Pb 2170 Å spectral line on a Techtron Model AA-5 atomic absorption spectrometer fitted with a grooved premix burner (Techtron AB-51) for air/acetylene, a Pb hollow cathode lamp (A.S.L.) operated at 5 mA, and with an aspiration rate of 5 ml min^{-1}. Readings to 0·001 in absorbance were obtained from a Techtron DI-30 Digital Indicator Unit in the averaging mode.

Particulates were collected on tapes of an A.I.S.I. automatic air sampler with a flow rate of 400 l h^{-1}, using Whatman No. 4 paper. The exposed area is circular with a diameter of 2·6 cm.

Calibration curve

Standard solutions containing 0–5 μg of lead per ml in 0·25 N nitric acid (diluted from concentrated nitric acid, Baker Chemicals, BAR, ACS) showed strict linearity (FIG. 1). The sensitivity (concentration necessary to produce 1 per cent absorption) was 0·15 μg of lead ml^{-1}. The coefficient of variation at lead concentrations of 0·1, 0·25, 0·5, 1 and 5 μg ml^{-1} was found to be 16, 10, 5, 3 and 0·8 per cent respectively. These figures show that 0·04 μg ml^{-1} of lead (readings to absorbance 0·001 can be performed by means of the averaging digital indicator unit), corresponding in the given procedure to

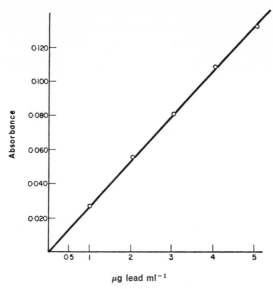

μg lead ml^{-1}

FIG. 1. Standard lead calibration curve.

0·1 μg m^{-3} of air, would have a coefficient of variation of nearly 40 per cent. BURNHAM (1969) reported a sensitivity of 0·25 μg ml^{-1} and coefficients of variation at 1 and 5 μg ml^{-1} of lead were found to be 19·3 and 3·7 per cent respectively.

Procedure for analysis of collected particulates

By means of a punching apparatus each spot (2·6 cm dia.) was cut out of the tape and placed in a 25 ml beaker, to which exactly 2 ml 0·25 N nitric acid was added by a dispenser. After waiting 30 min the absorbance was measured by spraying the extract into the flame and the result was directly converted on the digital indicator unit to μg of lead per cubic meter of air in the range of 0–12·5 ± 0·1 μg.

By spraying only 2 ml a steady reading can be obtained for samples with a low lead content (< 2·5 μg lead per spot). In cases of a higher lead content (dark spots) it is better to use 4 or 5 ml nitric acid.

When analysing spots of the A.I.S.I. smoke sampler by a chemical method (employing dithizone) a precision of only ±0·5 μg can be reached (CHOLAK, 1961).

The lead content of a blank filter (0·02–0·03 μg per spot or 0·01–0·015 μg ml^{-1}) could be neglected. BURNHAM (1969) found that the lead content of a glassfiber filter extract was 5 μg ml^{-1} at a volume of 8·8 ml.

The dissolution efficiency of particulate lead by 2 ml diluted nitric acid was tested by determining the lead content of ten already analysed (1–10 μg Pb), water washed spots. After complete oxidation with boiling HNO$_3$/H$_2$O$_2$ less than 5 per cent lead could be detected.

Matrix effects were tested by adding known quantities of lead to some filter samples; the results of recovery experiments by the proposed method are shown in TABLE 1.

From these figures it is evident that in contrast to the results of BURNHAM (1969) no reduction was found in the slope of the calibration curve owing to a matrix effect.

The usual dry ashing procedure, prior to analysis, was omitted here to maintain a simple routine method and because of the substantial resulting losses of lead (BURNHAM, 1969; LANDAU *et al.*, 1969).

BULLOCK and LEWIS (1968) also solubilize lead from smoke stains without ashing, as advocated by HANSEN, REILLY and STAGG (1965), prior to atomic absorption analysis of the nitric acid extract.

No interferences have been observed in the determination of lead by atomic absorption spectroscopy when an air–acetylene flame is used (ELWELL and GIDLEY, 1966). Even with phosphate no interference was found in the air–acetylene premix flame (SLAVIN, 1968).

The spots of dust on the tape were previously analysed by a reflectometer to determine the amount of standard smoke. It is of course necessary to avoid loss of material. In this manner no extra sampling equipment for the determination of particulate lead is needed.

199

TABLE 1. RECOVERY OF ADDED LEAD BY THE PROPOSED METHOD

Sample no.	Lead present (μg)	Lead added (μg)	Recovery of added lead (μg)
5	5·9	25·0	25·3
6	8·0	25·0	24·8
7	0·6	2·0	2·0
8	0·6	1·0	1·0
9	0·8	2·0	2·0
10	0·8	1·0	1·0

RESULTS

Over 8000 two-hour samples (even hours), collected during 1968 and 1969 at about 150 m WSW from Highway 13 at Delft, were analysed, yielding values of less than 0·1–9·1 μg of lead per cubic meter of air. The pattern of the two-hourly lead concentrations, plotted in FIG. 2 for the period 8–14 December 1968, reflects morning and afternoon rush hour traffic as well as meteorological conditions.

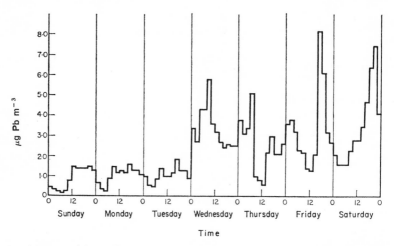

FIG. 2. Pattern of the two-hourly lead concentration during 8–14 December 1968 near Delft.

(In this period the wind direction varied from NE to SE; the first three days it was cloudy and near freezing point, during the last four days the weather was sunny and freezing.) More statistical results and correlation with meteorological data are reported in Research Report G 400 and G 406 of the Research Institute for Public Health Engineering TNO (in Dutch).

DISCUSSION

Atomic absorption spectroscopy together with the A.I.S.I. automatic air sampler provides a rapid, simple, precise and sensitive technique for two-hourly monitoring of the particulate lead content of the atmosphere. Tedious dry ashing and wet chemical procedures are found to be unnecessary, and by automating some steps hundreds of samples a day can be analysed.

HIRSCHLER and GILBERT (1964) and SNYDER (1967) have demonstrated that the organic lead content in ambient air is extremely low. Most of the lead in exhaust gas is in the form of inorganic particulate solids composed of lead halide (HIRSCHLER et al., 1964).

200

The results of two years form only a part of a long-term study to establish trends and levels in the concentration of atmospheric lead. Other heavy metals currently being investigated in our laboratory by atomic absorption are iron, zinc, cadmium and vanadium.

Acknowledgement—Thanks are due to G. BERGSHOEFF for critical examination of this manuscript.

REFERENCES

BULLOCK J. and LEWIS W. M. (1968) The influence of traffic on atmospheric pollution, *Atmospheric Environment* **2**, 517–534.

BURNHAM C. D., MOORE C. E., KANABROCKI E. and HATTORI D. M. (1969) Determination of lead in airborne particulates in Chicago and Cook County, Illinois, by atomic absorption. *Environ. Sci. Technol.* **3**, 472–475.

CHOLAK J., SCHAFER L. J. and STERLING T. D. (1961) The lead content of the atmosphere. *J. Air Pollut. Control Ass.* **11**, 281–288.

DIGGS D. R., HESSELBERG H. E., LUDWIG J. H. and MAGA J. A. (1963) Program for the survey of lead in three urban communities. *J. Air Pollut. Control Ass.* **13**, 228–232.

ELWELL W. T. and GIDLEY J. A. F. (1966) *Atomic-Absorption Spectrophotometry*, 2nd edn. p. 96, Pergamon Press, Oxford.

HANSON N. W., REILLY D. A. and STAGG H. E. (1965), *The Determination of Toxic Substances in Air*, p. 156. Heffer, Cambridge.

HELLER A. and KETTNER H. (1969), *Forschungsarbeiten über Blei in der Luft und Staubniederschlägen*, p. 55. Gustav Fischer Verlag, Stuttgart.

HIRSCHLER D. A. and GILBERT M. S. (1964), Nature of lead in automobile exhaust gas. *Archs Environ. Hlth* **8**, 297–313.

LANDAU E., SMITH R. and LYNN D. A. (1969) Carbon monoxide and lead—an environmental appraisal. *J. Air Pollut. Control Ass.* **19**, 684–689.

SLAVIN W. (1968) *Atomic Absorption Spectroscopy*, p. 120. Interscience Publishers.

SNYDER L. J. (1967) Determination of trace amounts of organic lead in air. *Analyt. Chem.* **39**, 591–595.

Sverre H. Omang

The determination of lead in air by flameless atomic absorption spectrophotometry

The determination of lead contents in atmospheric particulates by means of atomic absorption spectroscopy has been reported by several investigators[1-5]. In the usual sampling technique for such inorganically bound lead, the atmosphere under test is allowed to pass through some sort of filter in order to collect all particles above a certain size. The filter types used comprise glass fibre[4-6], filter paper[7] and millipore filters[1]. After the absorption, the filters can either be treated directly with hydrochloric acid[5] or nitric acid[6] or they can be dry-ashed at $500°$[4,7]. These methods have stood the test of experience and are very useful. However, large volumes of air must be aspirated through the filters to obtain enough lead for a determination. This makes the sampling rather time-consuming or requires heavy high-capacity pumps.

When peak values or instantaneous values are of interest, aspiration times of 10–15 min or shorter and much smaller equipment are desirable. The new graphite furnace technique introduced by L'Vov[8] in 1963 and further developed by Massmann[9], West and Williams[10], Donega and Burgess[11] and Welz and Wiedeking[12], has recently been marketed as a commercially available unit. This offers a unique possibility of determining trace elements in extremely small volumes with a high degree of accuracy. Since many samples can be injected into the graphite tube without a prior digestion or preconcentration step, most of the usual contamination encountered in ordinary trace element·analysis is avoided.

The present communication describes the use of this technique in a simple, rapid and extremely sensitive method, combined with collection of lead particulates on millipore filters from air volumes down to 10 dm^3.

Equipment and reagents

Air contaminants were collected on 37-mm diameter MF-Millipore filters AA (0.8 μm), made of mixed cellulose esters. These filters were connected to a small portable battery-operated pump (Casella, London), calibrated to 2.7 dm^3 air per min.

A Perkin-Elmer Model 303 Atomic Absorption Spectrophotometer equipped with a Perkin-Elmer (Bodenseewerk) Graphite Cell HGA 70, an automatic recorder readout accessory and a Hitachi–Perkin-Elmer Recorder Model 159 was used. Small sample aliquots were injected into the graphite tube by means of Eppendorf Marburg micropipettes. Flame atomic absorption measurements were carried out on a Perkin-Elmer 403 Atomic Absorption Spectrophotometer with a Boling burner head. A lead Intensitron hollow-cathode lamp was used as light source in all measurements. The only chemical used, nitric acid, was of analytical-reagent grade quality.

Lead solutions. A 1000-p.p.m. stock solution was prepared from 1.000 g of pure lead metal dissolved in 25 ml of nitric acid and diluted to 1˙1 with distilled water. From this solution 0.1-p.p.m. standard solutions containing 5 ml of nitric acid per 100 ml were prepared daily.

Measurements conditions

Before sample volumes are atomized in the graphite tube, any solvent, organic material or other unwanted components of the matrix must be removed. Smoke signals or false absorption will otherwise occur. Therefore, two separate heat treatment stages, drying and charring ("ashing") must be carried out before the atomization step. For such treatment, the HGA 70 is equipped with seven fixed programmes for easy reproduction of selected temperatures between 60° and 1100° and three clocks for time adjustment. The final atomization temperature is determined by the voltage for the resistance heating of the tube.

Since there is little available information about the settings of the instrument for each type of analysis, the optimal time and temperature of the various stages had to be determined. It was found suitable to dry the sample at 100°, to char at 330° and to atomize at 1900°. Program 4 and a transformer setting of 5 V (2.5 kW) takes care of this automatically. A period of 30 sec for each sequence was found satisfactory.

Procedure

Collect particulate lead samples by aspirating air for 10 min through the millipore filters. Soak the filters in 2.0 ml of 1 + 1 nitric acid in a 50-ml beaker and apply gentle heat. After 5 min, decant into a 10-ml volumetric flask and wash the filters with successive 2-ml portions of warm distilled water. Finally dilute to volume with distilled water.

Inject 5–50 μl of 0.1-p.p.m. lead standard solution into the graphite tube and register the lead absorption peak at program 4 with a 5-V atomization voltage and a 30-sec sequence time. Prepare a blank solution from a new millipore filter treated with nitric acid as described above and register a blank value. Prepare a calibration curve from the peak height measurements after converting percentage absorption to absorbance and subtracting the blank value. (A straight line is obtained up to 2 ng of lead.) Measure small sample volumes in the same way, convert the peak heights to absorbance, subtract the blank value for the same injection volume and evaluate the lead concentration from the calibration graph.

Light scattering

Light scattering, causing too high absorption readings, is well known in flame absorption measurements. Such interference can be corrected for by selecting a non-absorbing line within 10 nm of the analytical line and subtracting the absorption signal from the analytical value. It was found necessary in the present work to examine the peaks for such unspecific absorption. The analytical line used was 217.0 nm and the non-absorbing line was 209.8 nm. In the regular sample and standard solutions, no absorption was recorded at 209.8 nm. In order to establish if the lead particles had been completely dissolved and washed out of the millipore filters, the filters were treated with 1 ml of hot nitric acid; the filters dissolved completely and the solutions were diluted to 10 ml. For the same aliquot sizes (20 μl), the same signals (11%) were recorded at both lines. This was taken as evidence of light scattering and also of complete lead extraction when the millipore filters were leached as recommended in the procedure.

Results and discussion

The proposed method was used in the analysis of a number of air particulate samples collected in Oslo city in November 1970, 1 m above street level. Some of the results obtained are shown in Table I. It is obvious from these data that the sampling and analytical methods used offer satisfactory sensitivity. With 10-min sampling times and 20-μl injection volumes, the sensitivity obtained for 1% absorption is about 0.7

TABLE I

ANALYSIS OF STANDARDS AND SAMPLES OF OSLO CITY AIR

(Scale expansion 1)

Sample	Air volume (dm^3)	Aliquot (μl)	Peak height (% abs.)	Total amount[a] (ng)	Concentration in air $(\mu g\ Pb\ m^{-3})$
0.1 p.p.m. standard	—	5	14.4	0.5	—
0.1 p.p.m. standard	—	10	24.4	1.0	—
0.1 p.p.m. standard	—	20	41.5	2.0	—
Blank	—	20	1.9	0.07	—
Blank	—	100	9.2	0.35	—
Air sample 1, rush hour	27	20	12.2	0.43	7.9
Air sample 2, rush hour	27	20	17.5	0.66	12.2
Air sample 3, rush hour	27	20	6.5	0.18	3.3
Air sample 4, suburb	54	100	10.1	<0.05	< 0.2

[a] Corrected for blank lead content.

μg of lead per m^3 air. The injected volume can easily be increased to 100 μl. This was done in air sample 4, but the high lead content in the analytical-grade nitric acid, determined to be 3.5 $\mu g\ l^{-1}$ makes it doubtful that a correspondingly better sensitivity can be assumed. For lead concentrations below 1 $\mu g\ m^{-3}$ of air, an increased sampling time or the use of less contaminated acid will give higher sensitivity.

The small sample volumes made it impossible to check the accuracy of the obtained analysis by preconcentration techniques and regular atomic absorption spectrophotometry. However, some sort of comparison was possible since the two solutions with the highest lead concentrations, sample 1 (22 $\mu g\ l^{-1}$) and sample 2 (33 $\mu g\ l^{-1}$) could be measured directly on the Model 403 with maximum scale expansion. The measured values of 26 and 37 $\mu g\ Pb\ l^{-1}$, respectively, are in acceptable accordance, when the low accuracy of the direct flame method in this concentration range is taken into consideration.

1 C. L. CHAKRABARTI, J. W. ROBINSON AND P. W. WEST, Anal. Chim. Acta, 34 (1966) 269.
2 G. THILLIEZ, Anal. Chem., 39 (1967) 427.
3 J. CHOLAK, L. J. SCHAFER AND D. YEAGER, J. Amer. Ind. Hyg. Assoc., 29 (1968) 562.
4 C. D. BURNHAM, C. E. MOORE, T. KOWALSKI AND J. KRASNIEWSKI, Appl. Spectrosc., 24 (1970) 411.
5 M. BEYER, Atomic Absorption Newsletter, 8 (1969) 23.
6 R. MOSS AND E. V. BROWETT, Analyst, 91 (1966) 428.
7 V. SMOLCIC, Arhiv Hig. Rada Toksikol., 17 (1966) 309; Anal. Abstr., 14 (1967) 5775.
8 B. V. L'VOV, Spectrochim. Acta, 24B (1969) 53.
9 H. MASSMANN, Spectrochim. Acta, 23B (1968) 215.
10 T. S. WEST AND X. K. WILLIAMS, Anal. Chim. Acta, 45 (1969) 27.
11 H. M. DONEGA AND T. E. BURGESS, Anal. Chem., 42 (1970) 1521.
12 B. WELZ AND E. WIEDEKING, Z. Anal. Chem., 252 (1970) 111.

Revision of a Field Method for the Determination of Total Airborne Lead

By D. M. GROFFMAN AND R. WOOD

THE field method for the determination of total airborne lead devised by Dixon and Metson[1] was later adopted by H.M. Factory Inspectorate Committee on Tests for Toxic Substances in Air and published by H.M. Factory Inspectorate in their booklet series[2] "Methods for the Detection of Toxic Substances in Air." It is the policy of this Committee to request that the Laboratory of the Government Chemist carry out periodic revisions of the field methods published in this booklet series.[3] This allows account to be taken of any changes in the threshold limit value of the particular toxic substance or even in its use within industry. Also, any procedural disadvantages in the test which have been shown up since it was first developed can be investigated and, if these are overwhelming, a new test can be devised. The lead test had been in existence for eight years and some experimental disadvantages had emerged in that time. This paper describes the modifications made to the test to obviate these.

EXPERIMENTAL

The original test[2] involved four stages: the collection of the airborne lead (dust or fume); the dissolution of the collected sample; the formation and extraction into carbon tetrachloride of the coloured lead dithizonate complex from a buffered (pH 11) aqueous solution; and, finally, the visual comparison of the colour obtained with a range of standard colours. Each stage was examined in this present revision.

COLLECTION OF AIRBORNE LEAD—

Millipore type AA membrane filters were selected. These have been recommended[4] as suitable for the collection of industrial fume samples and their use would bring the lead test into line with field tests for the determination of copper, iron oxide and zinc oxide fumes and dusts in industrial atmospheres, which are also being devised in this laboratory and which are to be published. There appeared to be no particular advantage in the use of either Whatman No. 2 or Munktell No. 00 filter-papers for collection of the sample as in the original method.[2]

A lead fume was generated by atomising aqueous lead acetate solutions and igniting the resultant aerosols formed in an apparatus that is to be described elsewhere.[5] It was found that the collection efficiency of the Millipore filters was constant at least over a range of 1 to 5 l minute^{-1} sampling rate. There was no reason to expect any variation from this when larger sized particles such as dusts were being collected.

DISSOLUTION OF COLLECTED LEAD SAMPLE—

It was found possible to dissolve the collected lead quantitatively from Millipore filters by soaking the filters for 5 minutes in the nitric acid - hydrogen peroxide solution originally used.[2] There was therefore no need, as in the original method, to decompose the filter to achieve dissolution.

The original test[2] based on the use of the reagent dithizone was considered, on the basis of eight years' experience, to be sufficiently sensitive and specific for the determination of lead at its threshold limit value[6] of 0·2 mg m^{-3} when a 15-litre atmosphere sample was taken. However, certain disadvantages had become apparent. These were the use in the test of the highly toxic solvent carbon tetrachloride (threshold limit value 65 mg m^{-3}),[6] the poor and variable keeping properties (only a few hours in some cases) of the carbon tetrachloride solutions of dithizone, the variable reagent blanks and responses to a standard amount of lead of different batches of dithizone, and the absence of a one-half threshold limit value colour standard.

Choice of organic solvent—Of the other chlorinated hydrocarbons that could be used, only 1,1,1-trichloroethane possessed a threshold limit value high enough (1 900 mg m^{-3})[6] to make the change from carbon tetrachloride worthwhile. In 1,1,1-trichloroethane solution it was found that the spectrophotometric response of lead dithizonate was increased by a factor of 1·2 compared with that in carbon tetrachloride under similar test conditions, the wavelength of maximum absorption being 520 nm. A slight disadvantage in the use of 1,1,1-trichloroethane was that it separated less clearly than carbon tetrachloride from the aqueous phase. However, this was easily overcome by running the organic phase through a strip of Whatman No. 1 chromatographic paper (20 × 80 mm) previously rolled up and inserted into the stem of the separating funnel. The inhibitors present in some of the commercially available brands of 1,1,1-trichloroethane tested, apparently comprising a number of compounds, appeared either to react with the dithizone producing yellow background colours or to decompose the dithizone so that insufficient reagent remained to complex the lead completely. The use of uninhibited solvent, which is available from some chemical suppliers, is therefore essential.

Dithizone reagent—While the original dithizone solution[2] (40 mg dissolved in 1 litre of carbon tetrachloride) was reasonably stable if it was shaken with a reducing solution, such as sulphur dioxide in water, and thereafter kept in a refrigerator, this was inconvenient for field use. At room temperature (20 °C) this solution was found to deteriorate markedly in a few hours. A more concentrated 1,1,1-trichloroethane solution of the reagent, 40 mg per 100 ml, was found to be considerably more stable at room temperature, the rate of deterioration being such that solutions up to 7 days' old could be used. In the field this stock solution required to be diluted ten times prior to use in a test. However, even by using this procedure the dithizone reagent blank, shown as a yellow colour, gradually increased with time such that the visual colour differentiations at the various concentrations of lead became difficult. Tests appeared to show that the production of the yellow blank was a temperature effect rather than a photochemical one. Removal of this yellow background colour from the 5 ml of 1,1,1-trichloroethane solution of dithizone to be used in a test, together with any coloured metal dithizonate complex blank that may have been present in the reagents, was found to be possible simply by extracting the dithizone solution in a separating funnel with the aliquot of buffer solution to be used in the test. The lower, organic, layer containing the coloured interferences was separated and discarded.

The buffer solution containing the dithizone reagent was retained in the separating funnel and to this was added the dissolved lead sample, followed by 5 ml of fresh 1,1,1-trichloroethane. (Since dithizone appeared to have a limited stability of a few hours in the alkaline buffer solution it was found desirable to pre-extract each aliquot of dithizone working solution just prior to its use). The lead dithizonate was then extracted into the 1,1,1-trichloroethane layer, which was run off, and its colour was compared with standards. The colours produced from 0 to 15 μg of lead were found to be stable for at least 3 to 4 days provided that the organic solutions were tightly stoppered. The dilute dithizone solution was usable for at least 8 hours after preparation provided that each aliquot was treated as above before being used in a test.

A survey of the different commercially available dithizone reagents indicated that several gave reduced colour responses with lead. Stock 1,1,1-trichloroethane solutions of such dithizone reagents also decomposed rapidly, usually producing a red instead of green colour. In view of this a simple sorting test was devised to preclude the use of unsatisfactory dithizone reagent in this method for lead. Details of the sorting test are given later in the method.

Buffer solution—With the introduction, as indicated above, of a preliminary extraction designed to remove any lead reagent blank, involving the aliquots of dithizone and buffer solutions that were to be used in the test, it was no longer found necessary to prepare singly the constituents of the buffer solution. The revised buffer solution (see section on Reagents) had a pH of 11.

Colour standards—The original test[2] had visual colour standards representing 0, 3, 6, 12 and 15 μg of lead, which corresponded respectively to 0, 1, 2, 4 and 5 times the threshold limit value when a 15-litre sample of atmosphere was taken. The disadvantage of this set of standards was the absence of a half threshold limit value. With the increased colour response obtained through the use of 1,1,1-trichloroethane instead of carbon tetrachloride, colour differentiation between the two highest levels became more difficult and it was decided in this revision to omit the original top level. It is now recommended that if test atmospheres are suspected to contain greater than four times the threshold limit value of lead a smaller sample than the normal 15 litres should be taken and the appropriate correction factor should be applied to the standards. With the increased colour response and lowering of reagent blanks observed with this revision, it was found possible to include a half threshold limit value standard. Details of the preparation of the colour standards are given below.

INTERFERENCES—

Although not departing from the main feature of the original method,[2] *i.e.*, the use of dithizone reagent for the determination of lead, it was considered prudent to re-examine the possible interference effects of other metals that might occur with lead in industrial atmospheres on this revised method. This was done by adding known amounts of these metals to solutions containing 1·5 μg of lead (equivalent to a 15-litre sample of an atmosphere containing half the present threshold limit value of lead) prior to the determination of the latter. Under the test conditions up to 3 μg of copper, 15 μg of antimony(III) or 6 μg of cadmium did not interfere. These amounts were respectively equivalent to those which would be present in a 15-litre sample of an atmosphere containing twice the present threshold limit value of the interfering metal. On a similar basis iron(III) and zinc interfered but the levels that were tolerated, 50 μg in each case, were considered to be sufficiently high to allow lead to be determined by the field test in all but the most exceptional circumstances without interference from iron or zinc. Tin(II) ions in solution at a concentration as low as 15 μg interfered strongly with the test. However, it was considered that tin trapped on a filter would not be extracted in sufficient quantity by the nitric acid - hydrogen peroxide solution to cause interference. This was confirmed when 60 μg of tin(II) and 1·5 μg of lead were spotted on to a filter-paper that was allowed to dry. An extraction was carried out, and the lead was determined, 1·45 μg of lead being recovered.

METHOD

APPARATUS—

Filter-paper holder—A holder that will take filter-papers of 25 mm diameter.

Filter-paper—Millipore type AA (0·8 μm), 25 mm in diameter, and strips of Whatman No. 1 chromatographic paper, 20 $\times$ 80 mm.

Sampling pump—A pump capable of drawing air through the filter-paper at a fixed rate of between 3 and 5 l minute^{-1}.

Separating funnel—This was 100 ml in capacity, having a PTFE stop-cock and a glass stopper.

Glass tubes for colour comparison—These were 13·5 mm in i.d. and had a capacity of 10 ml. (Tintometer Ltd., Salisbury, supply pairs of tubes suitable for use in conjunction with the Lovibond "1000" Comparator.)

REAGENTS—

All reagents should be of analytical-reagent grade when possible.

Nitric acid - hydrogen peroxide solution—Dilute 5 ml of lead-free concentrated nitric acid (sp.gr. 1·42) to 100 ml with water and add 0·2 ml of 30 per cent. w/v hydrogen peroxide.

Buffer solution—Dissolve 3 g of potassium cyanide, 6 g of sodium metabisulphite and 5 g of ammonium citrate in about 200 ml of water, add 325 ml of ammonia solution (sp.gr. 0·88) and dilute to 1 litre with water. (This solution is stable for several months if stored in a polythene screw-topped bottle.)

Standard lead solution—Dissolve 192 mg of lead nitrate in 1 litre of 0·1 N nitric acid to give a solution containing 120 μg ml^{-1} of lead. Dilute 5 ml to 200 ml with 0·1 N nitric acid to give a solution containing 3 μg ml^{-1} of lead.

1,1,1-Trichloroethane, containing no inhibitor.

(Solvents supplied by Hopkin and Williams Ltd. or Fisons Scientific Apparatus Ltd. were found to be suitable for use.)

Dithizone stock solution—Dissolve 40 mg of dithizone in 100 ml of 1,1,1-trichloroethane. Renew this solution after 7 days.

Dithizone working solution—Dilute 5 ml of the dithizone stock solution to 50 ml with 1,1,1-trichloroethane. Renew this solution after 8 hours. (The suitability or otherwise of any batch of dithizone reagent must be assessed prior to the use for test purposes of a working solution prepared from that dithizone. A suitable sorting test for dithizone reagent is given below.)

PROCEDURE—

Place a Millipore type AA filter-paper in the holder, attach the assembly to the pump and draw a 15-litre sample of air through the paper at a rate of 3 to 5 l minute^{-1}. Disconnect the holder from the pump, remove the paper and place it in a small beaker not less than 25 mm in diameter. Add 2·5 ml of the nitric acid - hydrogen peroxide solution and leave it to stand for 5 minutes.

Add 15 ml of the buffer solution to the separating funnel followed by 5 ml of the dithizone working solution. Stopper the funnel and shake it vigorously for about 15 s. Allow the mixture to stand until the layers separate, then run off the lower layer and discard it. Dry the inside of the stem of the separating funnel with a rolled-up piece of filter-paper and then insert into the stem a rolled-up strip of Whatman No. 1 chromatographic paper, 20×80 mm in size. Transfer the acidic solution from the beaker to the funnel, wash the beaker with two 1-ml aliquots of water and add the washings to the funnel. Add 5 ml of 1,1,1-trichloroethane to the mixture, stopper the funnel and shake it vigorously for about 15 s. Allow the mixture to stand until the layers separate, run the lower layer into a colour comparison tube and compare the colour, preferably in daylight, with each of the lead colour standards contained in similar tubes. View the respective liquids against a white paper background.

SORTING TEST FOR DITHIZONE REAGENT—

Carry out the procedure (as above) from the stage at which 15 ml of buffer solution is added to the separating funnel up to, and including, the insertion of the rolled-up strip of paper into the stem of the funnel. Then add 2 ml of the dilute standard lead solution (3 μg of lead ml^{-1}) to the funnel. Add 5 ml of 1,1,1-trichloroethane to the mixture, stopper the funnel and shake it vigorously for about 15 s. Allow the mixture to stand until the layers separate, run the lower layer into a colour comparison tube and compare the colour, preferably in daylight, with the 0·4 mg m^{-3} of lead colour standard (see Table I) contained in a similar tube. Again, view the liquids against a white paper background. Unless a good match in both colour and intensity is obtained, the dithizone working and stock solutions should be rejected and fresh solutions should be prepared with a new batch of dithizone reagent. (If a spectrophotometer is available, an optical density of 0·36 $\pm$ 0·02 should be obtained in the sorting test by using a 10-mm cell and reading at 520 nm against a 1,1,1-trichloroethane blank.)

TABLE I

VOLUMES OF COBALT SULPHATE, COPPER SULPHATE AND POTASSIUM DICHROMATE SOLUTIONS PER 25 ml TO PRODUCE AIRBORNE LEAD FIELD TEST COLOUR STANDARDS

Lead standard/mg m^{-3}			0	0·1	0·2	0·4	0·8
Yellow component/ml	..	..	0·70	0·20	0·25	0·20	0·20
Blue component/ml ..	..	..	0·00	0·05	0·10	0·60	0·50
Red component/ml ..	..	..	0·20	1·00	2·80	5·50	10·20

The various components were added as follows: red component, dissolve 10 g of cobalt sulphate heptahydrate ($CoSO_4.7H_2O$) in 85 ml of water; yellow component, dissolve 0·1 g of potassium dichromate in water and make up to 100 ml; and blue component, dissolve 10 g of copper sulphate pentahydrate ($CuSO_4.5H_2O$) in water, add 1 ml of concentrated hydrochloric acid and make up to 100 ml with water. Prepare the colour standards by mixing these solutions in the proportions shown in Table I, diluting each to 25 ml with water and mixing throroughly.

As an alternative to the above colour standards, a series of permanent glass standards on a comparator disc was prepared in collaboration with, and is available from, Tintometer Ltd., Salisbury.

DISCUSSION AND APPLICATION OF THE METHOD—

Although designed specifically as a field test and not intended for the accurate determination of lead in air, this method can be used to determine lead accurately if a spectrophotometer is used. The required calibration graph can be prepared by using standard lead solutions and reading the intensities of the lead dithizonate colours in a 10-mm cell at 520 nm against a reagent blank.

The sampling technique in this revised method, apart from a change in the filter used, had not been materially changed from the adequately tested original.[2] Consequently, a detailed evaluation of sampling procedure was not considered necessary for this present work. However, by using samples of lead dust collected in an industrial atmosphere, trials were carried out primarily to check on the efficiency of dissolution of dust samples (compared with laboratory-generated and collected fume samples) collected on Millipore type AA filters. A wide range of sample weights was deliberately obtained by sampling volumes of the atmosphere considerably in excess of the normal 15 litres taken in the proposed field test. After carrying out the usual field test extraction the filters were decomposed by wet combustion and any lead present was determined. Table II shows that over a range of weights of lead, 2·2 to 62 μg in the dusts collected, the percentage extraction of the metal was independent of the weight and also entirely satisfactory for field test purposes. Table II also indicates that with a spectrophotometric finish the scope of this test can be extended to cope with larger samples of lead than can be determined using the visual colorimetric finish.

This work was carried out on behalf of the Department of Employment and Productivity Committee on Tests for Toxic Substances in Air. We thank the Government Chemist for permission to publish this paper and H.M. Factory Inspectorate for arranging facilities for the field tests.

TABLE II

EFFICIENCY OF EXTRACTION OF LEAD DUST SAMPLES FROM FILTERS
BY USING THE PROPOSED FIELD TEST PROCEDURE

	Lead found*/μg		
Sample	By extraction† of filters	By wet combustion‡ of extracted filters	Efficiency of extraction, per cent.
1	2·2	0	100
2	2·3	0·35	87
3	4·0	0·40	91
4	4·9	0·15	97
5	16·0	0	100
6	18·6	0·9	95
7	19·0	0	100
8	52·0	0·25	100
9	53·6	0·25	100
10	62·0	0·8	99

* By spectrophotometric version of field test procedure.
† With nitric acid - hydrogen peroxide solution.
‡ With fuming nitric acid - perchloric acid mixture.

REFERENCES

1. Dixon, B. E., and Metson, P., *Analyst*, 1960, **85**, 122.
2. Ministry of Labour, "Methods for the Detection of Toxic Substances in Air, Booklet No. 14, Lead and Compounds of Lead," H.M. Stationery Office, London, 1962.
3. "Report of the Government Chemist, 1968," H.M. Stationery Office, London, 1969, p. 99.
4. Farrah, G. H., *J. Air Pollut. Control Ass.*, 1967, **17**, 738.
5. Marshall, B. S., Telford, I., and Wood, R., in preparation.
6. "Threshold Limit Values 1969," Technical Data Note 2/69, Department of Employment and Productivity, London, 1969.

A Field Method for the Determination of Lead in Glass Used for Shielding Television Receiver Components

HARRY LEVINE and PAUL S. RUGGERA

Introduction

THE TRANSMISSION OF X-RAYS through the glass envelopes of certain types of television tubes, or through the glass covering x-ray fluoroscopic screens, is influenced by the amount and type of high-atomic-number elements in the glass. Interest in this aspect of the subject was stimulated by recent findings[1] that color television receivers have been shown to emit x-radiation in excess of NCRP recommendations,[2] particularly under certain conditions of operation and construction. These emissions have been found to originate from picture tubes, shunt regulator tubes, and high-voltage rectifier tubes.[3]

When conducting inspections of equipment where transmission of x-radiation is in question, it is useful for the inspector to know the composition of the glass so that its ability to absorb x-rays may be estimated. Of particular interest would be such items as the glass envelope of the shunt regulator rectifier and direct-viewed cathode-ray picture tubes used in color television receivers, and glass covering diagnostic x-ray fluoroscopic screens. One can detect substitution of nonleaded glass inappropriate for shielding by means of this test, rather than to perform an x-ray transmission measurement. Additionally, it is sometimes desirable to check the manufacturer's statement on the composition (particularly the lead content) of glass components, as these have been found, on occasion, to have been in error.

Lead is the element most commonly used in glass for its radiation attenuation, although barium is often used in the television picture tube face plate because it causes less coloration and loss of light transmission. A rapid, semiquantitative method for the detection and estimation of lead in glass, suitable for use in the field, has been developed. It is based on the action of a mixture of hydrofluoric acid and sodium iodide on lead contained in glass and ceramics.[4] Important features of this test are that the reaction can be

211

evaluated in a matter of minutes in the field without causing visible damage to the specimen, and the conventional chemical analysis that is generally performed in the laboratory can be eliminated. It will show at once whether lead is present in appreciable amounts or is essentially absent.

Dilute hydrofluoric acid is used to dissolve a small section of the glass to be tested and is left in contact with the glass surface for a minute or less. After the lead is detected, the acid can be washed away before any damage is done to the specimen. The reaction on the glass specimen produces a colored compound distinctive of lead even in the presence of small amounts of other metals such as barium, calcium, copper, manganese, iron, nickel, or chromium, some of which might have been added to the molten glass in order to introduce color. Glass samples tested showed 0% to 50% lead.

Preparation of Reagents

The dilution is performed by mixing 1 volume of 48% hydrofluoric acid with 3 volumes of distilled water to make 12% hydrofluoric acid. Add 0.005 gm of sodium iodide to each milliliter of diluted hydrofluoric acid to prepare the final reagent. The reagent may be kept indefinitely in a stoppered polyethylene bottle in the dark. The faint yellow color that might form owing to liberated iodine will not interfere with the test. The specimen to be tested should be perfectly clean and dry; the surface should be horizontal and the testing carried out on a bench or table adjacent to a sink with running water. Always keep the reagent in polyethylene containers, as hydrofluoric acid attacks glass. Bottles containing the reagent should be opened for only a minimum time necessary to carry out the test. Care should also be taken not to expose the skin to splashes of the acid or its vapor. Any acid inadvertently spilled must be washed away with a large volume of water at once.

Procedure

Apply one drop of the reagent on a convenient spot of the specimen with a polyethylene dropper and observe any color changes or precipitation. On curved surfaces, a small circle of silicone grease will enclose the drop and minimize spreading. If a considerable amount of lead is present, there will be an immediate precipitate of yellow lead iodide in the test drop. If only a trace is present, 2% or less, the drop will remain clear for a second or two and then a buff to yellow turbidity will form. A confirmation test that the yellow precipitate is lead iodide can be obtained by washing the yellow precipitate into a polyethylene beaker and adding to the washings a few crystals of NaI or KI. The yellow precipitate of lead will dissolve, giving a colorless liquid. If the specimen is a lime glass and has no lead, a white precipitate of calcium fluoride will appear on the surface.

An approximate estimate of the lead content was made by comparing the intensity of the yellow precipitate with standards. The speed of development and the depth of color are a guide to the amount of lead present. The standards were prepared from powdered samples of glass containing known amounts of lead. The powder was spread over the surface of a circular alumina disk having an area of 1 cm^2 and a thickness of 1 mm (Coors Porcelain Company, Golden, Colorado). The disk was prepared by coating it with a thin film of a 5% Aerosol OT solution (75% Aqueous) and then spreading 80 mg of the glass powder over the wetting agent. Percentages of the various glass powders ranged from 0% to 50% PbO. The alumina disks were placed in a cold muffle furnace, and the temperature was raised to 800°C. This temperature was maintained for 10 minutes, and then the disks were allowed to cool. A smooth glaze over the entire surface of the alumina disk resulted. Each alumina button was treated with one drop of the reagent, placed in an oven at 105°C for 10 minutes, and then cooled to room temperature.

The reagent produces a slight hazing of the surface of lime glass specimens, and a spot on the specimen that is not optically important should be used for testing. Different glasses show different resistance to attack by the reagent, depending on their composition. As the PbO content of the glass is increased, the SiO$_2$ and CaO content are decreased, while the Na$_2$O and Al$_2$O$_3$ content generally remain constant.

Discussion

Table I presents a comparison of the estimated amount of lead using the reagent drop method and the amount of lead determined by conventional methods in the various glass specimens analyzed. The lead content of the glass envelope in the various shunt regulator tubes was determined by atomic absorption spectrophotometry.[5]

The chemical composition of the various glass specimens is listed in Table II. The major constituents of the glass specimens were determined gravimetrically[6] and by atomic absorption spectrophotometry.[5] These data show the relationship between the lead content and other major constituents, such as silica. The silica content of the glass sample is decreased considerably when the lead content is increased. Several shunt regulator tubes, of both the earlier and the more recent version, were investigated to evaluate the usefulness of the lead determination described in this manuscript, in determining a relative correspondence between the amount of lead present in a glass envelope and the resultant x-ray emission from the tube. The tubes were used to expose four 14-inch × 17-inch film packs made up of a KK-type and a commercial-type film (Eastman Kodak Type SO142, Type SO125, Duo-Ready Pack, Rochester, New York). The film pack was formed into a 17-inch-high cylinder. When the cylinder was placed around the tube, the distance from the tube center line to the film was approximately 5 cm. Exposure was made at 30,000 volts and 0.5 mA for a period of 6 hours. The film was then developed under controlled conditions (new chemicals, constant temperature, gas burst agitation) so that exposure rate could be determined by using a densitometer and a set of calibration curves which relate density to exposure rate. The calibration of the film pack was performed by a free air ion chamber.

Table I

A Comparison of Lead Content in Glass Specimens Determined by Conventional Methods and by the Reagent Drop Method

Sample Identification	Determination by Conventional Methods (% PbO)	Approximate Estimation by Reagent Drop Method (% PbO)
Corning glass tube envelope (E-1)	26.47[a]	25
Corning glass tube envelope (E-2)	Trace[a]	0
#3720 TV picture tube safety panel (SP-1)	0[a]	0
#3755 or 3770 TV picture tube safety panel (SP-2)	4.87[a]	5
Corning 9019 TV picture tube face plate	Trace[a]	0
G.E. 6EH4 (GEH-020)	30.32[b]	30
G.E. 6EL4 (OWE-006)	30.52[b]	30
Sylvania 6BK4C (EMP-006)	50.06[b]	50
G.E. 6EL4 (OWE-117) new type	50.35[b]	50

[a]Determined gravimetrically.
[b]Determined by atomic absorption spectrophotometry.

Table II

Chemical Composition of Glass Specimens Used in Color TV Receiver Components

Sample Identification	PbO	SiO_2	CaO	MgO	BaO	Al_2O_3	Fe_2O_3	K_2O	Na_2O
Corning glass tube (E-1)	26.47	55.41	0.26	0.19	0.0	1.65	0.22	$K_2O + Na_2O = 11.72$	
Corning glass tube (E-2)	Trace	72.96	5.01	3.39	0.0	1.93	0.42	$K_2O + Na_2O = 16.45$	
#3720 TV picture tube safety panel (SP-1)	0	68.90	7.32	2.75	0.0	3.08	0.10	$K_2O + Na_2O = 16.82$	
#3755 TV picture tube safety panel (SP-2)	4.87	70.69	6.42	3.60	0.0	$Al_2O_3 + Fe_2O_3 = 1.67$		$K_2O + Na_2O = 12.43$	
Corning 9019 TV picture tube face plate	Trace	65.15	4.75	1.41	6.56	$Al_2O_3 + Fe_2O_3 = 5.49$		$K_2O + Na_2O = 16.49$	
G.E. 6EH4 (GEH-020)	30.32	55.21	<0.01	<0.01	0.0	2.46	0.45	10.28	3.68
G.E. 6EL4 (OWE-006)	30.52	56.42	0.0	0.0	0.0	1.36	0.0	9.38	3.16
Sylvania 6BK4C (EMP-006)	50.06	37.28	1.22	0.04	0.0	3.36	0.01	8.62	1.28
G.E. 6EL4 (OWE-117) new type	50.35	37.31	2.14	1.06	0.0	1.33	0.08	7.42	0.74

213

TABLE III
Relative Comparison between Lead Content of Glass Envelope
and Resultant Exposure Rate

Tube Type	Average Envelope Thickness (inches)	Chemical Analysis (% PbO)	Fast Method (% PbO)	Net Density of KK Film from Anode Beam	Exposure Rate (mR/hr)
G.E. 6EH4 (GEH-020)	0.035	30.32	30	3.78	11.7
G.E. 6EL4 (OWE-006)	0.050	30.52	30	1.10	3.33
Sylvania 6BK4C (EMP-006)	0.034	50.06	50	0.12	0.30
G.E. 6EL4 (OWE-117) new type	0.047	50.35	50	0.01	0.04a

aThis value was determined by extrapolation of the calibration curve.

Table III presents a comparison between the amount of lead present in the glass envelope and its influence on exposure rate. Increasing the lead content between the two thinner glass envelopes of tubes 6EH4 and 6BK4C reduced the exposure rate by a factor of 40. The other variable, the wall thickness of the envelope, also had some effect. When the 6EH4 is compared with the 6EL4, a reduction factor of 3.5 is observed. Cross comparisons with the new 6EL4 were not made, since a density of 0.01 is not a point on the calibration curve, and the exposure rate was estimated by extrapolating the curve to that value.

In summary, the field test for lead content of the shunt regulator tube could be a valuable tool in field surveys of sets found to emit excessive radiation. When a field of radiation is detected in the area of the shunt regulator tube, the investigator cannot be sure of the exact source, since it could be the shunt, the high-voltage rectifier, or the picture tube. Using the test kit, he can determine, with relative certainty, the lead content of the shunt regulator tube. If the tube contained approximately 50% PbO, then it could be eliminat⌐ᵈ as the defective component. This leaves the high-voltage rectifier, which is always in a metal cage for voltage protection and the picture tube. Since instrumentation is available by which one can determine the beam area, the elimination of the shunt regulator from consideration will almost certainly pinpoint the defective component. The picture tube will most probably have a large area beam, whereas the high-voltage rectifier would emit a beam only through the air holes in the cage and, therefore, be much smaller in area. A similar set of criteria can be set up for components other than the shunt regulator tube to deter.nine the relative comparison of x-radiation to lead content.

References

1. *X-Ray Protection Standards for Home Television Receivers*, Interim Statement of the NCRP (February 23, 1968).
2. National Council on Radiation Protection and Measurements (NCRP): *Radiology 75:* 122 (1960).
3. STEWART, H. F., *et al.*: X-ray Patterns and Intensities from High Voltage Shunt Regulator Tubes for Color Television Receivers. *Radiol. Health Data Rept. 8:* 12, 675 (December 1967).
4. KING, J.: *Museums J. 56:* 281 (March 1957).
5. JONES, A. H.: Analysis of Glass and Ceramic Frit by Atomic Absorption Spectrophotometry. *Anal. Chem. 37:* 1761 (1965).
6. Analysis of Glass, *Scott's Standard Methods of Chemical Analysis*, 5th ed., Vol. 2, p. 2164, Van Nostrand, Princeton, N. J. (1939).

A SIMPLE DEMOUNTABLE HOLLOW-CATHODE TUBE FOR THE ANALYSIS OF SOLUTIONS
APPLICATION TO LEAD IN BIOLOGICAL MATERIALS

N. J. PRAKASH AND W. W. HARRISON

The hollow-cathode excitation source introduced by Paschen in 1905[1] has found increasing use in recent years for the emission spectroscopic trace analysis of metals and non-metals[2-4]. This highly energetic, controllable excitation source has been shown to yield better sensitivity for many elements[5], particularly non-metals. The rapid development in the field of atomic absorption spectroscopy has contributed considerably to the revival of interest in the hollow-cathode excitation source.

The analysis of solutions by this technique presents certain difficulties owing to the low pressure environment of the hollow-cathode tube. A few investigators[6,7] have reported such solution analyses, including an earlier study from this laboratory[8]. In the present investigation, a shielded graphite cathode which is suitable for analysis of the acidic residue from wet-ashed biological materials is described. To facilitate such analyses, a very simple demountable hollow-cathode tube assembly has been constructed which allows a stabilized discharge, high emission intensity, and a short turn-around time. Characteristics of this hollow-cathode excitation system are demonstrated for standard solutions and biological samples.

EXPERIMENTAL

Hollow-cathode source

The demountable hollow-cathode tube previously used[8] was quite suitable for emission analysis but subsequent experience with the hollow-cathode excitation technique indicated that design improvements could be made, including simplification. Construction of the previous tube was laborious, the numerous vacuum-seal points presented potential leak sites, and the cathode was not directly accessible for cooling. The tube design used in the present investigation is shown in Fig. 1. The stainless steel cathode holder block was machined to mate with a 40-mm i.d. glass joint (Kontes Glass Co.), with a Viton O-ring and pinch clamp for the vacuum seal. A brass water jacket (solder connection) permitted water cooling of the cathode holder block, as well as the graphite cathode assembly which could be slipped into the cathode holder cavity. The demountable stainless steel anode was attached to the glass envelope with a 0.25-in Cajon Ultra Torr fitting, and the front of the glass tube was sealed with a quartz optical grade window using silicon rubber. The discharge was localized between the anode and cathode cavity by shielding the cathode holder block with a center drilled quartz disc flush against the holder and a 1.5-in diameter glass shield which extended over the cathode–anode interspace. The cathode–anode distance was normally set at about 1 cm. Compared to the previous tube, the present tube can operate at high currents, owing to the water cooling capabilities. Our power supply was limited to 200 mA capacity, but higher currents could be used with no damage to the tube. A higher signal-to-background ratio was also observed, but increased ease of operation was perhaps the greatest advantage.

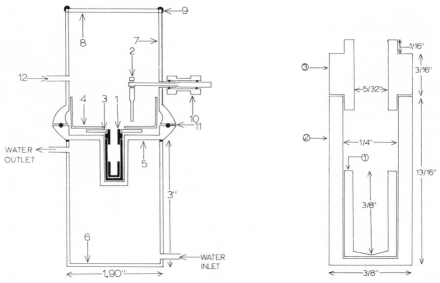

Fig. 1. Demountable hollow-cathode source showing (1) graphite cathode assembly, (2) stainless steel demountable anode, (3) quartz disc shield, (4) outer glass envelope shield, (5) stainless steel cathode block, (6) brass water jacket, (7) O-ring vacuum glass connector, (8) quartz window, (9) Silicone rubber seal, (10) Ultra Torr vacuum connection, (11) Viton O-ring, and (12) gas inlet.

Fig. 2. Graphite hollow-cathode assembly showing (1) inner electrode (sample receptor), (2) outer graphite electrode, and (3) graphite assembly cap.

The assembled hollow-cathode tube was used in both the horizontal and vertical modes. The latter was more convenient with respect to shield placement and access to the cathode cavity, as well as general ease of demounting, and was used for all the data reported here. The water-jacketed cathode holder was kinematically mounted on a 65-mm Ealing Tri-Rack flat-bed carrier which was movable along an Ealing 500-cm triangular steel optical bench. A front surface mirror mounted at a 45° angle to the vertical hollow-cathode tube directed the emission radiation through two quartz focussing lenses and into the spectrometer. The spectrometer, readout, and vacuum system have been previously described[8].

Hollow-cathode assembly

The cavity in the stainless steel cathode holder was intended to accommodate many different types of cathodes, including those of pure metal to act as a line source for atomic absorption. For the analysis of solutions, possibly of small volume, the assembly shown in Fig. 2 was used. The outer graphite electrode acts as a housing which fits into the holder cavity. The smaller inner electrode contains the sample deposition and, upon ion bombardment, allows the production of an atomic vapor which is advantageously concentrated within the assembly by the bayonet friction fitting cap. The inner analytical electrode was discarded after each run, but the outer graphite electrode and cap could be used for 10–15 runs before significant background from residual amounts of the trace test element appeared.

Reagents

All chemicals used in this study were reagent-grade. The graphite hollow-cathode assemblies were machined from "Ultra Purity" spectroscopic grade electrodes (Ultra Carbon Corporation, Bay City, Mich.). Standard solutions were prepared by dilution of Fisher atomic absorption standards. The laboratory distilled water was further purified by passage through a mixed ion-exchange bed and used for dilution of standards and final rinsing of glassware.

Procedure

A series of standard solutions of the analyte was prepared, each containing an added carrier salt concentration of 1000 p.p.m. lithium and 500 p.p.m. potassium. The small inner graphite cathodes were dip-coated with collodion over the entire extra-cavity surface to prevent the loss of test solution by diffusion through the porous graphite. The treated electrodes were air-dried, followed by the addition of 0.1-ml increments of the test solution which were dried under an infrared lamp. Four such increments were normally used. The cathode with the dry residue was heated for a few minutes in a muffle furnace at 450° to destroy the collodion coating, to expel any last traces of water, and to aid in degassing the graphite.

The electrode was then transferred to the larger graphite electrode and the assembly inserted into the cathode block. After tube assembly and evacuation, the system was flushed with argon filler gas, re-evacuated, and filled with argon to a pressure of 35 mm oil (16 mm oil = 1 mm Hg). The discharge was initiated at low currents and quickly increased to the 200-mA working current. The low p.p.m. and sub-p.p.m. concentrations of test element produced a pronounced emission maximum, subsequently falling off to background within minutes. Blanks were run for each sample to determine any background contribution caused by carrier salt, cathode, or sample treatment. Experimental parameters such as wavelength, slit width, current, and fill gas, were optimized in preliminary studies with standard solutions.

RESULTS AND DISCUSSION

Problems related to solution analysis

The transition from solution sample to a test element film deposited in the cathode cavity requires the consideration of several factors. An inert, pure metal hollow cathode with a simple emission spectrum would seem ideal as a deposition site, but this may depend upon the salt content of the solution. In a sample containing no particularly high elemental concentrations, the deposited sample film will normally cause no discharge problems, but small changes in major component concentration may significantly alter the analyte discharge environment with a subsequent change in test element emission intensity. Conversely, a high salt content which allows a certain spectroscopic tolerance in the concentration variation of major constituents may produce a sample film which essentially acts as an insulator either to prevent discharge initiation or at least to create erratic behavior. Graphite, as a hollow-cathode medium, has several advantages. It is obtainable in high purity, in many physical forms ranging from blocks to powders, and has a relatively simple emission spectrum.

A further significant advantage of graphite is the fact that it is unaffected by acidic or basic solutions that could seriously react with various metals. Initially an attempt was made to use a suitably drilled graphite rod as a receptor for the solution sample, but the porosity of the graphite transmitted the solution through the rod, resulting in sample loss. Pressed graphite pellets, with the sample solution applied dropwise and dried on the pellet surface, were then used but the high carrier salt content created discharge stability problems. The next approach was the formation of a homogeneous slurry of the sample solution and graphite powder which was dried and pressed into a pellet for analysis. A stable, reproducible discharge resulted, but in addition to reduced sensitivity, the inconvenient and time-consuming preparation step was a marked disadvantage. The method as finally evolved makes use of collodion-coated thin-wall graphite electrodes which prevent sample diffusion out of the electrode but do not cause all of the carrier salt to deposit as a non-conducting surface layer. With this arrangement, it was possible to produce uniform elemental sensitivities with a minimum of pretreatment steps.

Spectroscopic buffer

In an earlier investigation[8] a carrier salt was used to impede the loss of test element from the cathode cavity during discharge by producing a more even and controlled volatilization. In applying the method to biological samples, the high concentrations of sodium and potassium, which may vary from sample to sample, caused changes in analyte emission intensity. The alkali halide carrier salt content which could be tolerated with stainless steel electrodes was not sufficient to provide a constant sample matrix. However with the graphite electrodes, it was discovered that a very high added carrier salt concentration of up to 5000 p.p.m. in the sample solution still allowed a stable discharge. This was used to advantage by preparing various combinations of alkali halide salts to act as both a carrier salt and a spectroscopic buffer to negate the variation of intrinsic concentrations of these species in biological samples. Best results in terms of precision and buffer action in the presence of variable sodium and potassium concentrations, were obtained with a stock solution from which each sample solution was made to be 1000 p.p.m. in lithium chloride and 500 p.p.m. in potassium chloride.

Studies with lead solutions

Working solutions of lead at the low p.p.m. range were used to optimize experimental parameters, including choice of filler gas, gas pressure, and tube current. The 405.8-nm emission line provided the best combination of sensitivity and freedom from interference. All solutions contained the previously described carrier salt. The emission response of a lead solution in the hollow-cathode discharge is shown in Fig. 3 along with a blank comparison of the carrier salt.

218

The ability of the method to eliminate problems caused by variation of sodium and potassium was of particular interest since the method was to be eventually applied to biological samples. Test solutions of lead plus carrier salt were doped with increasing amounts of sodium and potassium from 0 to 400 p.p.m., a concentration

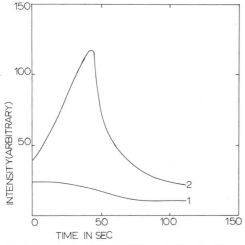

Fig. 3. Emission response of 405.78-nm lead line for (1) cathode-carrier salt background and (2) a 0.20 p.p.m. standard lead solution with added carrier (1000 p.p.m. lithium, 500 p.p.m. potassium in solution). Filler gas, argon at 35 mm oil (16 mm oil = 1 mm Hg); slit width 0.05 mm; tube current, 200 mA.

which was expected to be beyond the upper limit to be encountered after digestion and dilution of the biologicals. The carrier salt seemed to act as an effective discharge saturation buffer, because repeated test measurements showed no significant change in lead emission as the alkalis were added. The variation to be encountered in real biological samples would normally be less than these extreme conditions and should be effectively neutralized.

Lead in biological materials

Lead is of obvious interest in biological samples. Although lead is almost always present in tissues, its concentration is quite low, leading to digested samples in which lead is at the sub-p.p.m. level. This may impose serious sensitivity requirements unless concentration steps are taken, such as extraction. Hollow-cathode excitation was used to establish a working curve from lead standard solutions to cover the 0–1 p.p.m. range, with a limit of acceptable accuracy and precision ($\pm 6\%$) encountered at the 0.1-p.p.m. level.

Samples of human hair and cat liver tissue were analyzed for lead by the described method after wet digestion by a procedure previously described[8]. Table I shows the values obtained for the hair samples and tissue samples. Dry sample weights ranged from 0.2–0.5 g with a dilution after digestion to 5 or 10 ml in a volumetric flask.

In order to define more clearly the accuracy and efficiency of the technique for these sample types, recovery studies were made to determine the effect of the digested sample on lead emission. Aliquots of a digested sample were taken with increasing amounts of lead added, followed by emission analysis of each. Two hair samples and one liver sample were used with recovery values of 93.0, 99.5, and 92.3 % obtained.

TABLE I

LEAD ANALYSES IN THREE DIFFERENT HAIR SAMPLES AND ONE LIVER SAMPLE AS DETERMINED BY HOLLOW-CATHODE EXCITATION

Sample	Lead concentration ($\mu g \ g^{-1}$, dry wt.)
Hair III	4.10
Hair II	8.10
Hair	7.03
Liver tissue	2.00

The biological analyses are presented not to suggest any particular significance of lead in these samples, but rather to show that the hollow-cathode excitation technique could be used to obtain such data from small portions of samples containing low lead concentrations. The very simple design of the demountable tube eliminates serious instrumental problems and allows stable operation. It has been very useful in our laboratory as a complementary technique to atomic absorption.

This work was supported by Grant No. GM-14569, USPHS.

REFERENCES

1 F. PASCHEN, Ann. Physik, 50 (1916) 901.
2 J. R. McNALLY, G. R. HARRISON AND E. ROWE, J. Opt. Soc. Amer., 37 (1947) 93.
3 G. MILAZZO AND N. SOPRANZI, Appl. Spectrosc., 21 (1967) 256.
4 K. THORNTON, Analyst, 94 (1969) 958.
5 J. A. PEVSTOV AND V. A. KRASILSCHIK, Zh. Analit. Khim., 21 (1966) 863.
6 G. L. STRIKENBROCKER, D. D. SMITH, G. K. WERNER AND J. R. McNALLY, J. Opt. Soc. Amer., 42 (1952) 383.
7 G. A. PEVSTOV, V. A. KRASILSCHIK AND F. A. YAKOVLEVA, J. Anal. Chem. USSR (English Transl.), 23 (1968) 1569.
8 W. W. HARRISON AND N. J. PRAKASH, Anal. Chim. Acta, 49 (1970) 151.

James W. Sayre, M.D.
David J. Wilson, Ph.D.

A Spot Test for Detection of Lead in Paint

Lead poisoning is one of the most important environmental health hazards in inner-city children today. The disorder almost always results from the child eating chips of paint, putty, or plaster containing toxic quantities of lead. Identification of painted surfaces which contain dangerous quantities of lead is an extremely important part of the household investigation in any case of lead poisoning. Furthermore, paint testing is a valuable means of locating potentially dangerous areas in homes where there are small children. Window sills, walls, and other interior surfaces are pointed out as particularly common sources of lead.[1,2] Heretofore, testing of paint samples by spectroscopic methods has been tedious, expensive, and required that specimens be submitted to a laboratory. A semiquantitative method suggested by Kaplan and Shaull,[3] while easier, still has the limitation of requiring technical ability, equipment, and dangerous chemicals. The method of testing herein proposed is simple, inexpensive, and specific, and can be performed in the patient's home. It involves the precipitation of lead as an insoluble black sulfide through the following reaction:

$$Pb + Na_2S \longrightarrow PbS$$

Method

A solution of sodium sulfide of about 5 to 8% is prepared. This solution must be kept tightly covered to prevent loss of potency through hydrolysis, which releases volatile H_2S. It is conveniently dispensed in 5 ml polyethylene squeeze-dropper bottles. Sodium sulfide does not attack the surface of these bottles. A label, "Poison: Harmful to Eyes or if Swallowed" is affixed. In this concentration there is no skin irritation, but the characteristic odor of hydrogen sulfide may persist on one's hands for a half-hour. While the total amount of sodium sulfide in this small bottle (250 to 400 mg) is of low potential toxicity,[4] it should nonetheless by kept out of the reach of young children.

The paint can be tested either in situ or as a full-thickness chip of paint removed from the surface of the wood or plaster. If testing is done in situ, it is essential that all layers of paint be exposed down to the bare surface by making a diagonal cut with a sharp penknife. If the paint is tested as a chip, a similar diagonal cut is needed so that all layers of paint may be wetted by the sodium sulfide solution. This is essential since the deeper, older layers of paint and particularly the primer coat may be the only ones which contain lead. Paint which has been more recently applied is less likely to contain hazardous amounts of lead. All layers should be inspected carefully for a color change (Fig. 1). Adequate lighting is most important for proper interpretation of the test, particularly when evaluating dark colored or soiled paints. At times a hand magnifying lens is very useful.

Sensitivity

This is a qualitative reaction and the intensity of the color change varies directly with the amount of lead present. Over the past 2 years in a lead paint screening program in Rochester, over 200 homes have been inspected. When the sodium sulfide testing method was introduced, chips were taken to the laboratory and examined with both sodium sulfide and spectroscopic methods. A black color developed in specimens proven to contain between 10 and 25% lead. However, quantitative determinations on specimens of paint composed of many layers may not yield an accurate comparison,

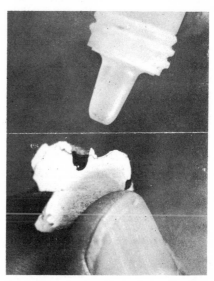

Fig. 1. Chip of paint with two layers. Top layer (toward camera) has turned quite black. Under layer is only slightly gray, indicating lead in range of 2 to 5%.

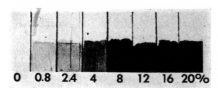

0 0.8 2.4 4   8 12 16 20%

FIG. 2. Gradations of color changes in paint of known lead content. Note light gray color has developed with paint containing less than 1% lead.

since all layers of paint are not necessarily lead-containing. For this reason, a specimen of exterior white primer paint of known composition was obtained from a local paint manufacturer. By calculation from the formula used in production, the paint contained approximately 22% lead in the wet state. A specimen was then dried and its lead content measured quantitatively. This resulted in a yield of 18% lead. Assuming the value to be approximately 20%, the paint was diluted with another sample of white paint known to contain less than 1% lead. Paint of successive dilutions was then applied to wood surfaces, dried, and tested with the sodium sulfide solution. Small wooden samples were pieced together and a comparator block made (Fig. 2). It can be seen that gradations of light gray through dark gray to black are obtained and that at the lowest dilution of 0.8% a faint gray color is present. Colors at the 15 to 20% range are dark enough to make it difficult to approximate lead concentrations over this amount.

Specificity

A host of other heavy metals may be found in paints. Those found in large quantity are zinc, titanium, and barium, none of which form black sulfides. Other metals are constituents of pigments and occur in amounts less than 1%: cadmium, chromium, cobalt, iron, manganese, magnesium, mercury, molybdenum, and nickel.[5] Of these, black sulfides are formed by iron, nickel, mercury, and molybdenum but the quantities present are small enough to cause no confusion. Copper also forms a black sulfide, but its only use in paint is for its anti-fouling properties. It would have no place in household paints. Black paint may be difficult to interpret, but is not ordinarily made with lead.[5] Care must be taken, however, in testing metal surfaces covered with paint such as pipes, or radiators since the iron or copper may be precipitated.

Discussion

Surveys made in a number of U.S. cities have demonstrated the prevalence of lead painted household interiors to be as high as 50 to 70%. To cope with so prevalent a condition as this, the use of expensive methods that require transport of samples to a laboratory or the use of other devices *in situ* may be out of the reach of health departments or other community groups. This method, however, when used as described herein, puts testing within the reach of many people such as public health nurses, community aids, and volunteers. A comparator block such as shown in Figure 2 is easily made and could be used as a standard if extensive testing was planned.

There are a number of other advantages offered by the sodium sulfide spot test:

(1) The method is simple, inexpensive and involves a minimum of chemicals and equipment. The small dropper bottle with its tight-fitting cap is easily carried in one's pocket or the glove compartment of a car. The bottles can be obtained from most pharmacies.

(2) Little training is needed in the interpretation of the color change. Care must be taken to test all layers of paint down to and including bare wood or plaster.

(3) The testing can and should be done in the home, particularly in areas accessible to children. Attention should be paid to areas where children have been observed to pick at walls or windowsills. Loose chips of paint on the floor or on the ground outside should also be tested.

(4) Testing may be done at the time surfaces are scraped and refinished. In several instances in Rochester the house painter was shown how to do this.

(5) The simplicity of performance and ease of interpretation has proven this spot test an adjunct to screening campaigns to identify early cases of lead poisoning.

Spectroscopic lead analyses were performed by Luville T. Steadman, Ph.D., Department of Radiation Biology and Biophysics of the University of Rochester, for which the authors are greatly appreciative.

REFERENCES

1. Chisolm, J. J., and Harrison, H. H.: The exposure of children to lead. PEDIATRICS, 18:943, 1956.
2. Barltrop, D., and Killala, N. J. P.: Factors influencing exposure of children to lead. Arch. Dis. Child., 44:476, 1969.
3. Kaplan, E., and Shaull, R. S.: Determination of lead in paint scrapings. Amer. J. Public Health, 51:65, 1961.
4. Thienes, C. H., and Haley, T. J.: Clinical Toxicology. Philadelphia: Lea and Febiger, 1964.
5. Brown R. A.: Personal communication.

AUTHOR INDEX

KEY-WORD TITLE INDEX